Grov
Beautiful
Teeth

Simple Strategies for Your Child to Have Perfect Teeth for Life

Estie Bav

First published by Busybird Publishing 2018

ISBN
Print: 978-1-925830-47-7
Ebook: 978-1-925830-85-9

Cover image: Kev Howlett, Busybird Publishing
Cover design: Busybird Publishing
Layout and typesetting: Busybird Publishing

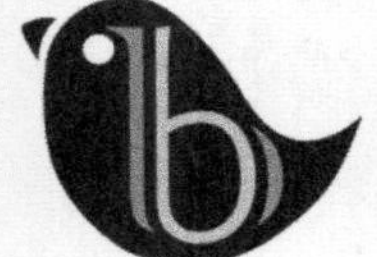

Busybird Publishing
2/118 Para Road
Montmorency, Victoria
Australia 3094
www.busybird.com.au

In loving memory of

my parents, who taught me the value of education

and my brother Frankie, who taught me about courage and resilience

Contents

Introduction

When I did my undergraduate training at the university dental school, my very first live patient was a kind and friendly 78-year-old lady who had lost all her teeth; I was learning how to make her a set of dentures, or false teeth. Subsequent patients for the rest of my clinical training were also adults in need of treatment to repair or to replace damaged or missing teeth.

Not surprisingly, I was good at tooth repair for adults when I graduated but felt quite inadequate about treating children. This insecurity prompted me to continue with postgraduate studies with the aim of filling this gap. I also had the good fortune of meeting a few colleagues in my early days in practice who advised me that graduating from university was just the start of this journey of becoming a good dentist … that I must keep developing my skills by attending as many seminars and conferences whenever possible. This I have not stopped to this day.

I began to appreciate the importance of understanding the cause of my patients' dental problems, as this would guide me to provide the best solutions for them. This continual search for wisdom and many years of practising dental care and treatment to patients led me to see that common everyday tooth problems often are the result of many layers of other health and structural issues, and many of which began early in a young child.

Many of my patients have become parents and even grandparents. They ask me questions regarding what they can do for the dental health of their children because they want the best for them, and for them to avoid having to go through some of the treatment they had to have. And so, there was no escape for me but to continue to learn and to search for the answers to their questions.

As a dentist working in a general dental practice, I get asked these questions routinely:

- When is best time for their child to see the dentist for the first time?
- Should I be concerned when I see the new, lower-front teeth crowded out (coming through behind the baby teeth)?
- Why are there gaps between my child's baby teeth?
- Is the overbite (covering of the upper-front teeth over the lower) ok?
- Why is my kid developing an underbite? Will it be ok?
- My child is still sucking the thumb. When should that stop?
- My child grinds his/her teeth so loud at night. What does that mean?
- Will my child need braces?

The goal of this book is to provide some answers to questions the reader may have.

When I explain to the parents the cause of the dental problems we see and what can be done about it, I often get the following reply, 'It all makes so much sense, but how come nobody had ever told us about it earlier?'

This book is not quite about how to prevent tooth decay; there are many resources available on that subject. It is also impossible to cover the whole and every subject of dentistry in one book. Rather, it is about the journey of preventative dental care for your child by ensuring that their teeth will have every possible chance of growing right and growing well and starting the journey much earlier – before any tooth has even erupted in the mouth, and aiming for a most perfect set of teeth by natural means as nature intended.

I feel that time is of the essence, that the knowledge should be open to the public, especially parents who want to and can apply much of the practice for their child **now**. There are many other avenues for continuing education in dental health for parents and young professionals alike, especially in these days of global social media and internet. I know parents can access a myriad of information on the internet.

It is my wish to give these parents a clearer insight, and to share with the reader my thoughts and experience based on my day-to-day practice and my own continuing professional learning over the many, many years.

1

Today's Dental Reality

You the readers are not the only people who know precious little about how teeth grow (develop). It may come as a surprise to you that many in the health professions have at best only a perception of the subject. Traditional teachings of preventative dental health present a rather limited view of simply preventing tooth decay and gum diseases by avoiding sweet, sticky foods and by improving brushing habits, and preventing breakdown from trauma by using a mouthguard.

Preventative dental health should be much more. In my practice, I meet parents who want to learn how to help their child grow teeth that are not crowded, teeth that fit in harmoniously with their jaw and face resulting in beautiful smiles, teeth that ultimately will not give them temporo-mandibular joint (TMJ) pain or attribute to airway problems later in life.

Parents aim to do the right thing for their children and are very proud that the kids clean their teeth well and have no cavities. But, do they know how the child's jaws need to grow to their maximum potential to allow plenty of room, not just for the teeth, but for the tongue and airway as well?

Today, many parents expect their child will need some orthodontics (braces) to straighten their teeth when their adult or second set of teeth come through. Many even accept that their child's beautiful and unblemished teeth will need to be sacrificed to deal with crowding. In our more affluent societies, it is common for children to undergo orthodontic treatment. Dental surgeries advertise their various offers of orthodontic services using tantalising names.

Dentists, like many other health professionals, tend to focus on fixing problems rather than addressing or treating the causes of problems, even with crooked teeth. This is what they are taught to do in their undergraduate years. When I was at university, the dental course focused on how to treat a patient's present problem, especially on how to repair teeth.

If the dental graduate goes out with the bachelor's degree and a practice license but does not seek to expand his or her knowledge beyond what was taught, then that will be all he or she is programmed to do: fixing and repairing damaged or unsightly teeth.

Traditionally, the patients also tend to have a certain expectation of dentists. They assume that dentists are trained to just repair, remove and replace teeth. Focusing on repair means that we are all in agreement to let the damage come first.

The good news is that there is a better way. Except for any damage caused by sudden trauma such as an accident, most dental diseases and tooth misalignments develop slowly over time. If we understand the cause and processes of the disease or disrepair, then we can take steps to stop or mitigate it.

When it comes to guiding the jaw and teeth to grow correctly and beautifully, most dentists tend to leave treatment until too late. The current trend is to let it grow awry and then come back to fix it in the best possible way at a most affordable point in time.

I want to show parents that it is simple to understand what may be causing these common dental problems. Once they understand what causes or influences growth issues, they will be able to prevent them right from the beginning. They will find that they do have much control over their child's growing set of teeth. Yes, parents have the power to take steps to prevent growth problems for their child. But they need to start early, the earlier the better.

You may be relieved to know that not all kids have to have 'orthodontics' or treatment using braces to correct crowding and crooked teeth. Children get crooked teeth because their jaws are underdeveloped (too small). If we understand what may be causing the underdevelopment, then we will be able to do something to encourage growth from an early age.

The need for orthodontic treatment was not common or even heard of in our ancestor's time. Admittedly, that could be due to a lack of know-how and resources. I was born and lived the first 15 years of my life in a country where having braces was unheard of.

Orthodontics still is uncommon or unheard of in many parts of the world. So, how come this has become so necessary in modern society? Perhaps orthodontics was not meant to be necessary. Until recently, there had been little need for the understanding of dental growth and associated problems. Our Palaeolithic ancestors did not need to seek this knowledge because their environment and culture gave them naturally beautiful straight teeth as nature intended. So, what did they do that is different from us? What was their culture and habit?

There are communities where tooth crowding and crooked teeth are not the norm. When I was working in a dental clinic at the World Trade Centre in Melbourne, I used to treat foreign workers and sailors who came off the ships that docked at Port Melbourne. They mostly sought emergency dental pain relief or tooth repair treatment during their stop-over. I was able to observe with interest and wonder that many of these men who came from far-flung countries have a full dental arch with hardly any crowding at all. They usually have kept all their teeth including their wisdom teeth.

In 2003, I got involved with a NGO and visited Vietnam where I provided free dental care to communities in the countryside. I observed that it seems to take only one generation for the change from having nice, wide jaws and uncrowded straight teeth to the next generation having crooked teeth. I observed that many of the children I treated aged about 11–12 years had crooked teeth, whilst their parents and teachers – a few of whom had tooth pain issues – had room in their jaws for all their adult teeth, beautifully aligned, including their wisdom teeth.

My observation is supported by the studies and observations made by a renowned dentist, Dr Weston Price, in the 1930s in the US. He wrote a book called *Nutrition and Physical Degeneration: A Comparison of Primitive and Modern Diets and their Effects.* He found that communities who are humming along happily with no issue of jaw and teeth alignment suddenly, within one generation, develop unattractive faces and crowded teeth when they adopted our so-called modern western diet.

However, I stress that there are several significant factors other than nutrition that can affect dental and jaw growth. Fortunately, there are now many studies done for a deeper, improved understanding of how teeth and jaw grow, and why and how this growth can go awry.

The reality is that we all admire people who have beautiful teeth and face, especially in our world of glamour and selfies. Looks have never been more important. The good news is that growing beautiful teeth, jaw, face and smile go hand in hand and can be a reality rather than just a dream.

At this point, I would like to explain to the lay person the various dental specialities and what the roles of each type of the dentists are.

A **general dental practitioner** or general dentist who has graduated with a bachelor's degree is qualified to practise all aspects of dentistry and is required to keep up with continuing education to ensure that they have the skill and competencies to provide dental healthcare for their patients. General dentists are usually the first port of call for a patient seeking dental treatment or advice.

In my practice, I would often be the parent's general dentist, sometimes having treated them for a long time. Now that they are becoming parents themselves, I always encourage the parent to bring the child in to say hello and to be familiar with the dental environment, the room, the sound, and what the dentist may do.

The best opportunity is when the parents are having their routine check-up. As a general dentist, I get to meet the child early in their life and I'm in a good position to look out for early signs of growth that may be heading in the wrong direction. I can advise parents how to initiate intervention as soon as the problems are detected.

I know of many general dentists like myself, who spend much time and resources keeping up with the latest in various fields, just so that they can provide the right type of advice even if they may not offer a particular service, or make appropriate referral to another health professional who does.

Dental specialists commonly relevant to children dentistry are pedodontists, orthodontists and oral surgeons. Although there are exceptions, specialists tend to keep to their chosen area of expertise and tend not to be interested in any other areas. They are technically very good in their own area of expertise and have obtained their qualifications through extra years of specialised training and examinations.

- **Orthodontists** are traditionally the specialists to go to for crooked teeth. They generally prefer treating older children because they are focused on aligning teenage/ adult teeth that have become crooked. They are especially skilled in using braces for tooth alignment.
- **Pedodontists** (also called **pediatric dentists**) specialise in the areas of tooth repair for young children and teens who may need special treatment. They are experienced at dealing with kids who have multiple tooth decay and who may often have behavioural issues that accompany treatment for these painful problems.

When there is an unusual injury or disorder of an individual tooth, the pedodontist would be the expert to go to. They usually have setups to provide treatment under general anaesthesia as required. If they detect that the child may be having tooth growth problems, such as crowding, then they are, traditionally, not supposed to deal with that issue directly. Usually, the pedodontist would then refer the child on to their specialist orthodontic colleagues for management.

- **Oral surgeons** (also known as **oral and maxillofacial surgeons**) are the 'nip-and-tuck' specialists dealing with surgery, and have excellent skills with scalpels, sutures, forceps and scissors, amongst others. So, wisdom teeth removal, especially when these teeth are impacted or stuck, will be the domain of an oral surgeon.

  When teeth and jaw development is totally out of whack, producing gross deformity of the face and bite, the oral surgeon may be called upon to cut the jaw and move the jaw segments for realignment and reconstruction.

Oral health therapists and/or hygienists are more specialised dental auxiliaries, many of whom can treat patients directly, although their range of responsibilities is not as extensive as a dentist's. They may further extend their education and training in the important and useful area of Orofacial Myotherapy.

Where do parents fit in? **Parents** are the obvious guardians for their child's dental health, starting from birth or even earlier. I suggest to parents to read this book right through, so they can understand what influences the growth and development of a child's teeth, to learn to recognise some simple signs of when teeth and jaw development are going wrong, and to learn how to take control and keep this growth along the right path early.

When parents take the best opportunities to do so early on, their child's teeth, jaw and facial growth will develop favourably and, furthermore, the child will gain many other health benefits.

2

Mouth: A Window to Health

Growing beautiful and healthy teeth is important. Teeth are part of the oral cavity, the opening for intake of food. It is obvious that teeth are important for biting off and chewing food, speech and communication, smile and other expressions, self-confidence and much more.

The act of eating, chewing and swallowing is normally taken for granted and we do not make any conscious effort to think about doing it. It is an awesome mechanism that involves more than just the teeth. Our teeth are part of a bigger system, the rest of the body in fact. It is for this reason that as a dentist, I need to pay attention to what I see in a patient's mouth beyond just their teeth.

When we take a bite of our food, our front teeth come together. The technical term for the connection of our teeth – that is, bringing the lower teeth to meet with the upper – is **occlusion.** The lay person word for occlusion is 'the bite'.

As we chew, the top (or upper) back teeth meet with the lower-back ones so that the bite-sized food can be broken and grounded down to make it easier to swallow and to release the nutrients for digestion. A **malocclusion** is when the top or upper teeth do not meet up with the lower teeth ideally, commonly described as having a 'bad bite'.

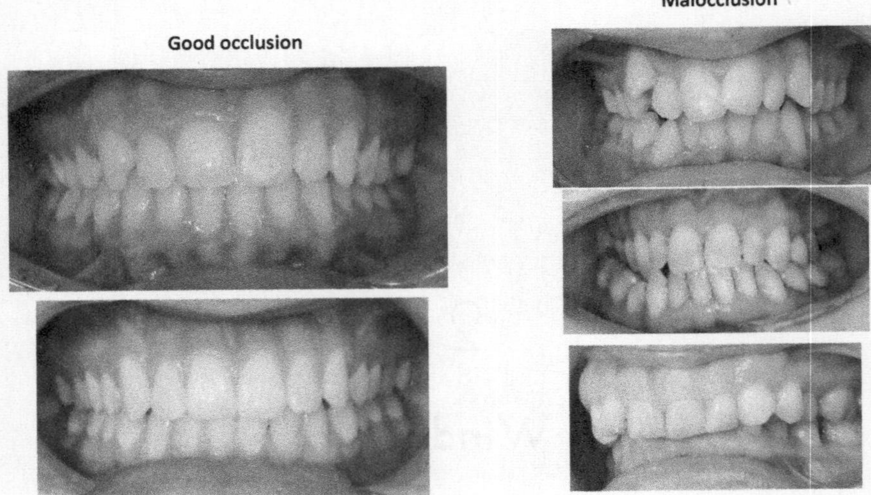

Figure 1: Good occlusion versus malocclusion.

Humans have two sets of teeth, the first set is called primary or deciduous teeth (the lay term is 'milk teeth') which erupt when the child is about 8–9 months old, and the last of these is usually lost at about 12 years old.

The second set is called secondary or permanent teeth (the lay term is 'adult teeth') which begin to replace the milk teeth when the child is about 6 years old. These gradually come through during the teenage years, with the wisdom teeth which are the furthest back and last molars to come through at the age of about 18 years or older.

There are 20 teeth in a full set of milk teeth, and 32 in adult teeth. Each set of teeth – be it primary or secondary – comprise of the incisors at the front for biting, cuspids or canines at the corners for gripping and tearing, and the back teeth or molars for chewing and grinding food.

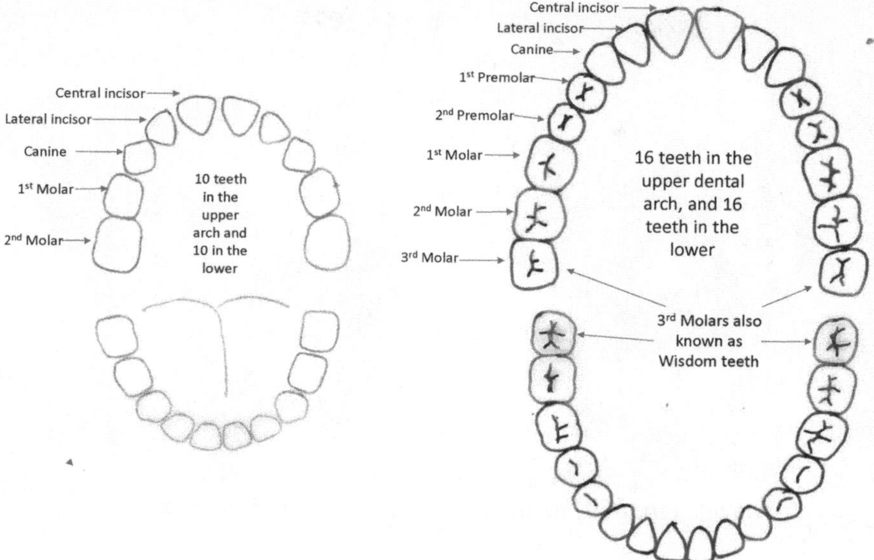

Figure 2: Primary and secondary teeth.

There are also the muscles which include the tongue and muscles of the jaw, the lips and cheeks. These muscles close the mouth and together with the tongue move the food around inside the mouth to make chewing possible before finally gathering the softened food to the back of the mouth for swallowing.

The bony part of the mouth to which the teeth are attached is the alveolar bone. The dental alveoli (singular alveolus) are the sockets into which the teeth are seated. The dental alveoli form part of the alveolar bone, which in turn is part of the jaw.

Whilst the lay person may think of the jaw as the lower jaw bone, dentists also refer the bony part of the mouth where the upper teeth are attached to as the upper jaw. The upper jaw is also commonly known as the **maxilla** and is made up of a pair of flat bones that join up along the midline to form the **palate** or roof of the mouth.

The border or rim of the palate is the upper dental arch formed by the upper teeth. The palate is part of the maxillary bone that connects with the base of the skull. The maxillary bone and all its parts form the midface or the middle part of the face.

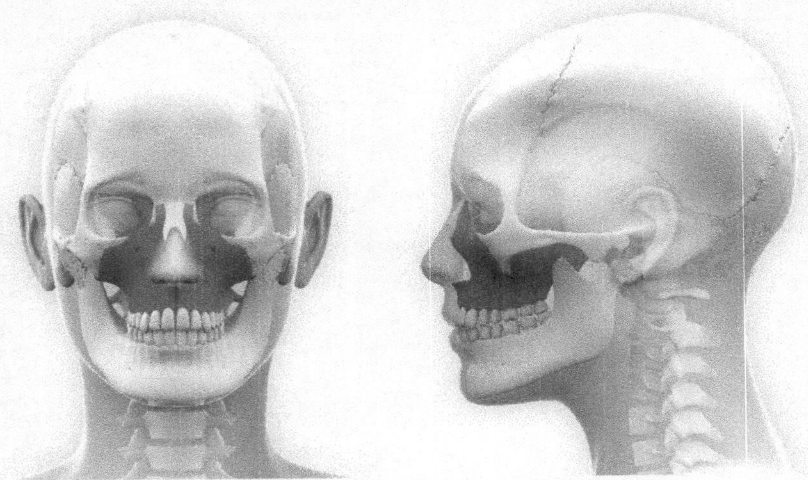

Maxilla (shaded) forms the nose, palate and midface

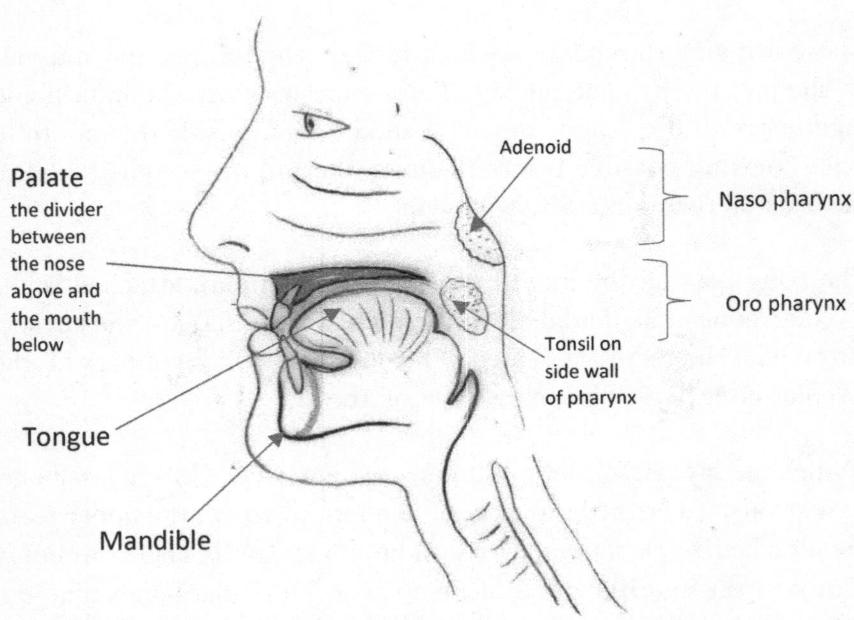

Figure 3: The maxilla.

The lower jaw bone is also known as the **mandible** and the lower teeth line up to form the lower dental arch. The mandible is a long bone that is horseshoe shaped, the two ends of which form the knob-like **condyles** that hinge with the base of the skull just in front of the ears. These two joints also known as the temporo-mandibular joints (TMJs) allow the various movement of the lower jaw against the upper jaw.

The TMJs are intimately related to the occlusion of the teeth, rather like a door which must fit closely within the door frame. One could see the TMJs as the hinges further back, whilst the occlusion forms the connection at the front – the door and the frame.

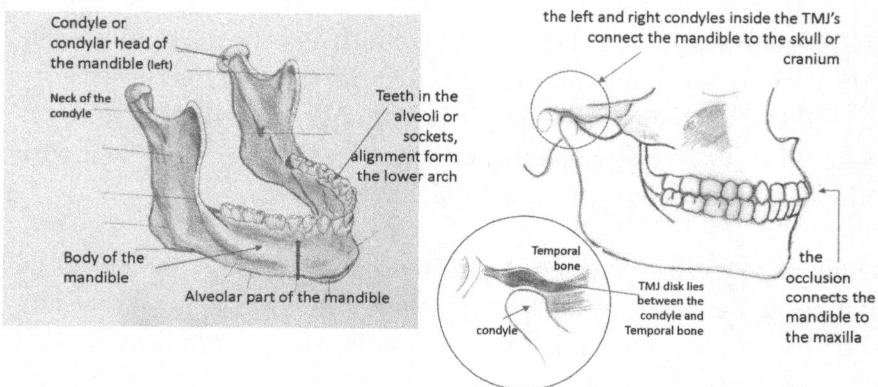

Figure 4: Mandible and TMJs.

The occlusion and the TMJs must function together harmoniously as they bring the lower teeth towards and close against the upper teeth, otherwise one or both will be stressed and can break down. TMJs are very susceptible to compression damage when teeth are not occluding optimally, when there is clenching and grinding of the teeth during sleep, and when the mandible and condyles are easily driven backwards by deflective inclines of the teeth.

Functional disharmony between them outside the very small limit of tolerance will create compression and a risk for dislocation of the condyle off the disk inside the joint. A repetition of such micro trauma will gradually lead to TMD.

Note that TMJ is often erroneously used as a term to describe TMJ disorders. The proper term for TMJ *disorder* should be TMD which stands for Temporo-mandibular Disorders.

The upper and lower dental arches need to be similar in shape and size so that the teeth can meet harmoniously to form a good occlusion.

The maxilla is connected to the base of the cranium or skull, whilst the mandible is hinged at the TMJs and its opening and closing movements are controlled by muscles and ligaments of the mandible, namely the masseter, the temporalis, the pterygoids and the various supra-hyoid muscles.

The palate is the divider between the mouth and the nose. The palate is the roof of the mouth and also the floor of the nose, or nasal cavity. It should be flat and wide. One of the common growth deformities is a vaulted and narrow palate, which forms a steep roof for the mouth and which encroaches into the nasal cavity above.

People with such a vaulted palate tend to also have narrow nasal cavities, a deviated nose septum, and a tendency for breathing difficulties through the nose. A narrow palate is commonly associated with crowding of the permanent teeth.

A steep palate will also restrict the proper posture of the tongue in the upper half of the mouth. The tongue should fit comfortably inside the palate when the mouth is closed. Refer to Figure 11.

The back of the mouth is the area of the throat known as the pharynx or more specifically the **oropharynx**. It sits just below the nasal pharynx which is the back of the nose. The pharynx is where the left and right tonsils and adenoids are located. It is important to appreciate the connection of these structures because, as you will see, growth and development can be affected by how the child breathes. Is the breathing routinely through the nose or through the mouth? Refer to Figure 3, page 10.

The dentist is the health carer who is in a good position to routinely check most of the above structures when the mouth is inspected. Sadly, dentists who are trained only to look at teeth will miss some very important and early clues related to health issues.

In other words, crooked teeth which are disconcerting can also alert us to how the surrounding structures – the palate, nose, mandible, tongue and other muscles – may have played a role and contributed to the crookedness. In turn, these can inform us how the child may be breathing or sleeping. Together with their surroundings, teeth can be tell-tale signs to the body's health. What we see in the mouth can tell us about how the child is breathing, eating, sleeping, feeling and how the child is growing.

I will discuss some common cases of malocclusions and what their teeth and occlusion can tell us about how the child's dentofacial growth and health. These are actual patients, but I have changed their initials to protect their privacy.

DI's Buckteeth

DI is an 8-year-old boy whose malocclusion displays a large dental overjet, meaning that the upper-front teeth project horizontally forward of the lower-front teeth. He also has a deep overbite: his upper incisors cover over the lower incisors almost completely.

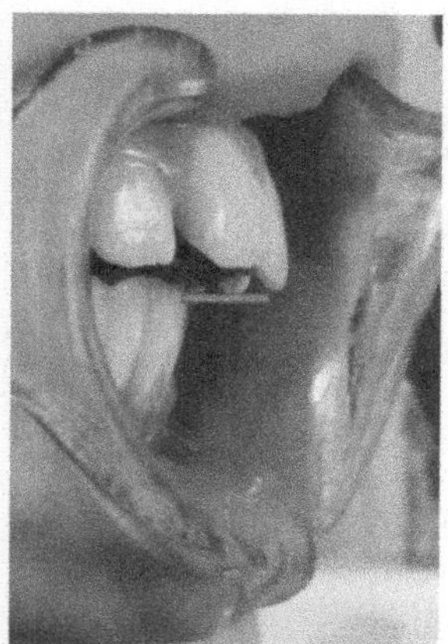

Overjet: horizontal

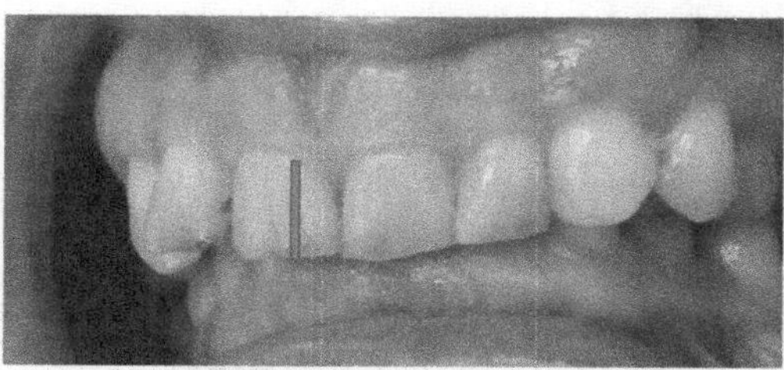

A deep over bite: 100% vertical overlap of upper incisors over the lower

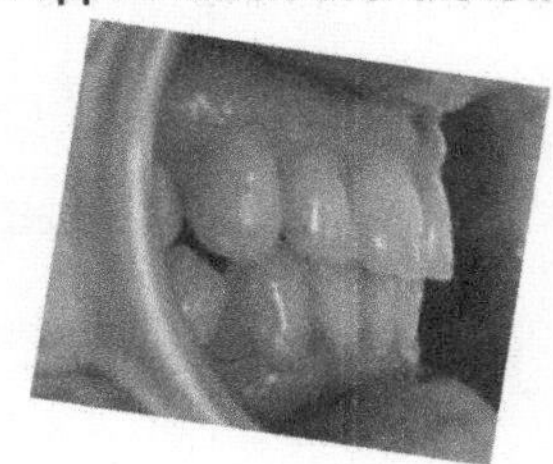

optimal amount of overjet/overbite

Figure 5: Overjet and overbite.

A large overjet is often a clue that there is a mismatch between the upper and the lower dental arches.

Usually, the fault lies in the maxilla not growing properly and may be too narrow at the front. When the upper dental arch is triangular in shape, it will not match the more rounded lower dental arch.

This situation often causes the mandible to position further back where the upper arch is wider, so the teeth can somehow occlude. An analogy could be that if the mandible is a foot trying to fit into a narrow, pointy shoe, then the foot cannot fit all the way to the toe of the shoe, thus leaving a gap in front of the foot.

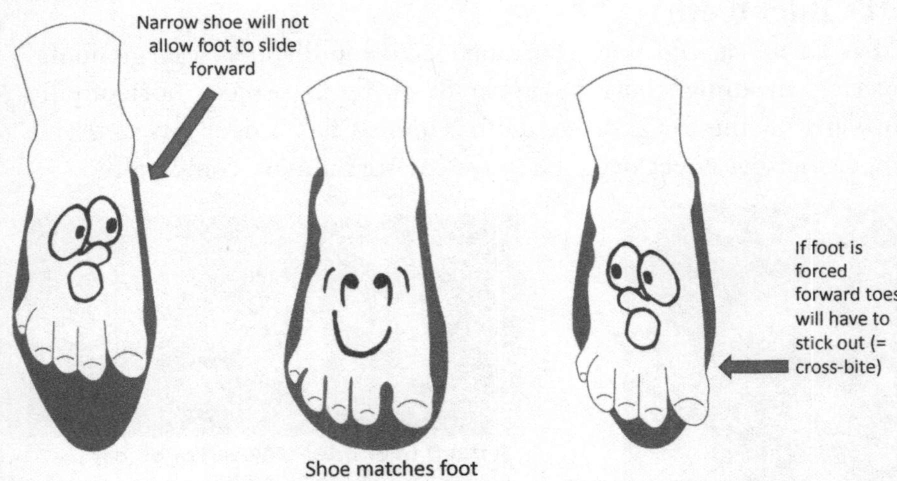

Figure 6: Mismatched foot and shoe.

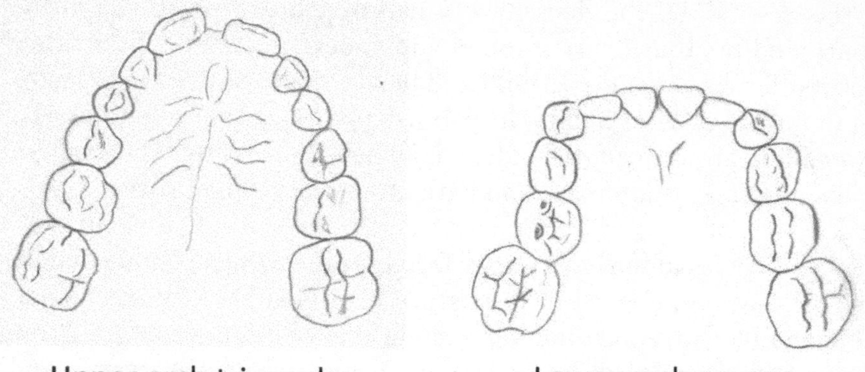

DI's arches can only fit together with the lower further back, forming a large overjet of his front teeth. He has a lowered tongue posture and poor oral musculature.

Figure 7: DI's mismatched dental arches.

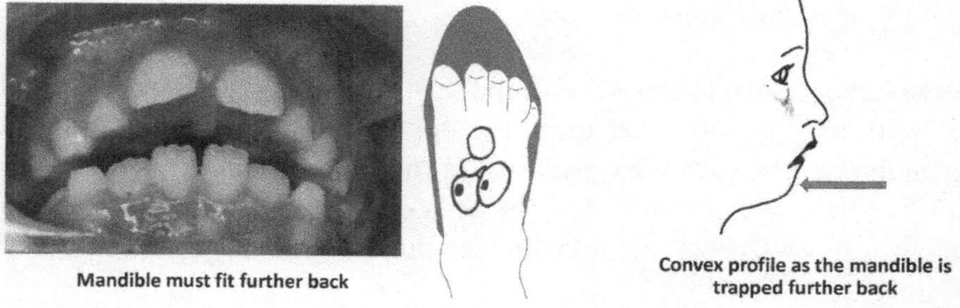

Mandible must fit further back
Convex profile as the mandible is trapped further back

Figure 8: DI's occlusion and facial profile.

The narrow upper dental arch gives us a clue that there is not enough room for the tongue to rest against the misshapen palate. In this situation, the tongue will rest in the lower half of the mouth and the mouth is more likely to hang open all the time. And when we see an open-mouth habit, we know that the child is breathing through the mouth and not the nose.

Furthermore, the child may be breathing poorly during sleep which will impact the quality of sleep. A whole string of other issues may result from disturbed sleep if we care to observe and investigate.

In the case of DI, he does have a habit of breathing through his mouth and his tonsils are swollen and appear inflamed. His mother reports that he often gets a cold and blocked nose which perpetuates the mouth-breathing habit. He also has poor facial muscle tone. His lower lip is always caught under his upper-front teeth. The corners of his mouth appear creased and are often cracked and sore.

DI also displays an unsatisfactory facial profile, which is immediately improved when he is asked to posture his mandible forward. When the mandible is trapped further back in the mouth and cannot grow forward, the condyles are at risk of being driven backwards and pressing against the sensitive nerve structures that are located at the back wall of the TMJs. We can predict that this child is at risk of developing TMD as he continues to grow without treatment.

HG's Constant Drooling

HG is a 5-year-old boy who is constantly drooling. His lips are always apart, and they look red and swollen. His open-mouth habit gives us a clue that the tongue must sit lower in his mouth instead of resting against the palate.

When the mouth is closed with the lips touching, we call that a good lip seal, but HG's lips are quite the opposite. His tongue will not be stimulating the palate to grow to its maximum genetic potential as it sits lower in his mouth and spreads out over the lower teeth. His occlusion is what we call an open bite caused by a tongue-thrust. (See Figure 27 in Chapter 6.)

His mother complains that he is a messy eater with food escaping from the corner of the mouth. This little boy needs to have orofacial myotherapy which is a mouth-and-tongue habit retraining program aimed at improving his chewing and swallowing by teaching him how to use his tongue and mouth muscles properly. (More details in Chapter 7.)

Simultaneously, his breathing needs to be corrected by maintaining a good lip seal and a return to breathing through his nose. Ideally, the mouth should be closed during sleep as well. HG's mother reports that he snores loudly during sleep, that he often has nightmares and sleeps poorly. The constant mouth opening tells us that he may have some blockages or obstruction in his nose or pharynx which may be preventing him from using his nose to breathe and that will need to be dealt with.

I referred HG to see an ENT (Ear Nose and Throat) medical specialist to investigate his nose and airway because, ultimately, we want him to be able to breathe through his nose so that he can keep his mouth closed and return the tongue to the correct posture against the palate.

When I reviewed HG two years later, I noted that he had not gone to see the ENT surgeon as advised. His mother explained that they have had been preoccupied with other health concerns: social and behavioural issues at school, and anxiety disorder. Scientists are currently investigating the connection between poor sleep and behavioural and learning issues in children.

BH's Tooth Clenching and Grinding

BH is a 7-year-old girl with signs of severe tooth clenching and grinding and tooth enamel wear. Her mother reports that she can hear BH grinding her teeth during sleep. BH displays a lot of gum when she smiles. Her front teeth lean backwards, her upper dental arch is flattened at the front instead of holding a nice rounded arch shape. Her tongue already appears to be very large for her mouth and she also carries an older look for her age, from a caved-in lower half of face.

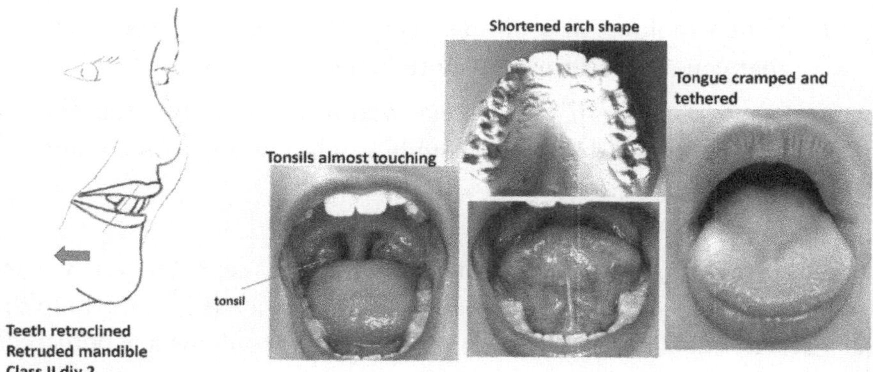

Her upper airway is compromised, and she clenches and grinds her teeth during sleep

Figure 9: Seven-year-old BH's teeth and related oral features.

Her symptoms as described above alert us to the possibility of an underdeveloped maxilla or midface which is not forward enough, inadequate airway with breathing issues. Her parents confirm that she sleeps poorly and she also snores loudly. Her tonsils are so large that they are almost kissing each other and are likely to be blocking her pharynx as well.

In addition to correcting her dental arch form to make room for her tongue and to create space for her permanent teeth to grow into, I referred this girl to see an ENT surgeon to assess her tonsils because it is vital for her to be able to breathe freely.

If her tonsils, airway and breathing issues are ignored, then she will not get the health benefits from good quality sleep that a child must have in order to grow to her best potential. If her upper dental arch is not developed to maximum potential, then her mandible will be trapped, and she is likely to have TMD symptoms as she continues to grow.

The three examples above show that:

1. There is a complex but important paradigm of mouth, jaw, teeth, nose breathing, sleep and growth that is at play which cannot be overlooked for maximum outcome and lifelong good health.
2. When looking at a child's teeth, we can easily see clues that can alert us to the way the child breathes.
3. The child's teeth, mouth, face and how he or she breathes and postures certainly provide a window into important health and growth issues.

Can it be too early or too late to tackle these issues? The answer is fortunately a resounding No, because all nature needs is some help to get growth back on track. But the earlier the problems are detected the easier it is to treat to perfection.

3

Beautiful Teeth for Life

We all know that in order to stay alive, we need food to provide nourishments and air to provide oxygen to every cell in our body. We can guess which of the two is of the higher priority by testing to see how long we can do without each one of them.

Just close your nose and mouth and hold your breath for as long as you can. Only a few minutes, right? It is always a priority for our body to get adequate air to stay alive, and not just any air but clean, good quality air that carries the right amount and proportion of oxygen. But air intake or breathing is something we tend to take for granted and not pay too much attention to.

Food and the nourishments just right for our body follow pretty closely behind on the priority ladder although far more attention is being paid to food as evident by the myriad of cookbooks, cooking shows on television and other doco-media, and endless discussions about dietary culture, philosophies and guidelines, and even age-old sayings such as 'You are what you eat'.

You may be wondering what have nourishments and **air** got to do with growing beautiful teeth?

A child will need to be breathing well and sleeping well in order to grow well, including the proper development of his/her teeth. This chapter explains why parents should be as focused on how the child is breathing as how the teeth are coming along. Growing beautiful teeth goes hand in hand with developing a wide jaw structure, forward midface and cheeks and a balanced and beautiful face.

When a child's face is growing in a forward direction and the mandible is also growing forward unhindered, the development of the bony structures provides plenty of space to allow teeth to grow straight and beautiful. This midface growth also provides for a clear nasal airway to facilitate breathing through the nose.

Children should be taught from a very young age and constantly reminded to breathe through the nose. Nature intends that we breathe through our nose and not our mouth. Babies are born nasal-breathers. Look around at newborns and you will observe that they keep their mouth closed and breathe through their nose even when they are sleeping. Yet we observe that at least half of the children around us revert to breathing through their mouth. Why? What happened to cause the change?

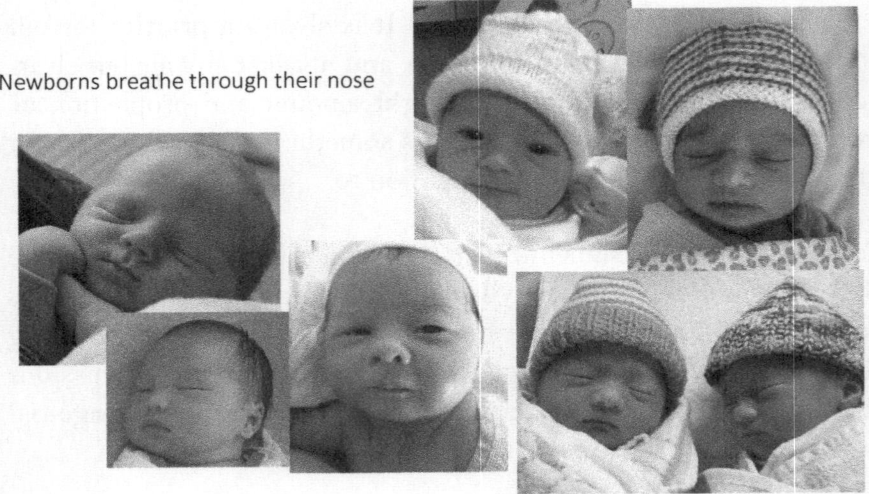
Newborns breathe through their nose

Figure 10: Natural nasal breathers.

Big Rewards for Breathing through the Nose

Inside the nose are structures called turbinates with a special lining that serves to prepare the incoming air. When we breathe in through the nose (and not the mouth), the air is filtered, warmed and humidified. In other words, the air is conditioned and just right for our body.

Breathing in through the nose also picks up **nitric oxide** (NO), a gas that is produced in the nose. This gas has antifungal properties and therefore sanitizes the air before it reaches our lungs. Nitric oxide is also essential for the exchange of oxygen at the cellular level. Therefore, having adequate oxygen intake in our breath isn't enough as we also need nitric oxide to facilitate the release of the oxygen molecules from the blood for uptake by the cells throughout the body.

Breathing in and out through the nose also maintains just the right volume of air passing in and out and reduces hyperventilating. To breathe through the nose, the child will need to keep the mouth held closed with lips lightly touching for a natural seal. This keeps the tongue nestled against the palate, which balances against the cheek muscles that press in from without.

Kids who breathe through their mouth tend to grow less attractive, longer and narrower faces and airway/breathing issues can accumulate through life. A child that always gets a snotty nose and who struggles to breathe through the nose is generally miserable, sad looking and less attractive except, of course, in the eyes of the parents. These kids tend to snore during sleep and parents would report that they are a poor sleeper and wake up suffering from foul breath due to mouth breathing.

Growing beautiful teeth, jaw and face is influenced by correct breathing through the nose – an ideal lifelong habit to adopt.

Tongue in the Palate

By keeping the mouth closed, it becomes easier to breathe through the nose, and this also keeps the tongue naturally held against the palate which is the key to maxilla growth.

Every time we swallow our saliva, the tongue should press into the maxilla. In a growing child, this contact stimulates the palate to grow broad and flat, producing a wide dental arch with ample room for the growing teeth. This also enhances the development of the nasal cavity to give plenty more space for air passage and stimulates midface growth in the forward direction. In other words, proper breathing habit, balanced facial growth and beautifully aligned teeth go hand in hand.

The three must go together: breathe through nose, lips touching, tongue resting against the palate with no deviant habit. Dr Steve Galella, a dental educator from Tennessee, referred to this as the 'Big 3'. It is so simple. When adopted at a young age, the Big 3 becomes natural and easy, and will stay with the child for amazing health benefits.

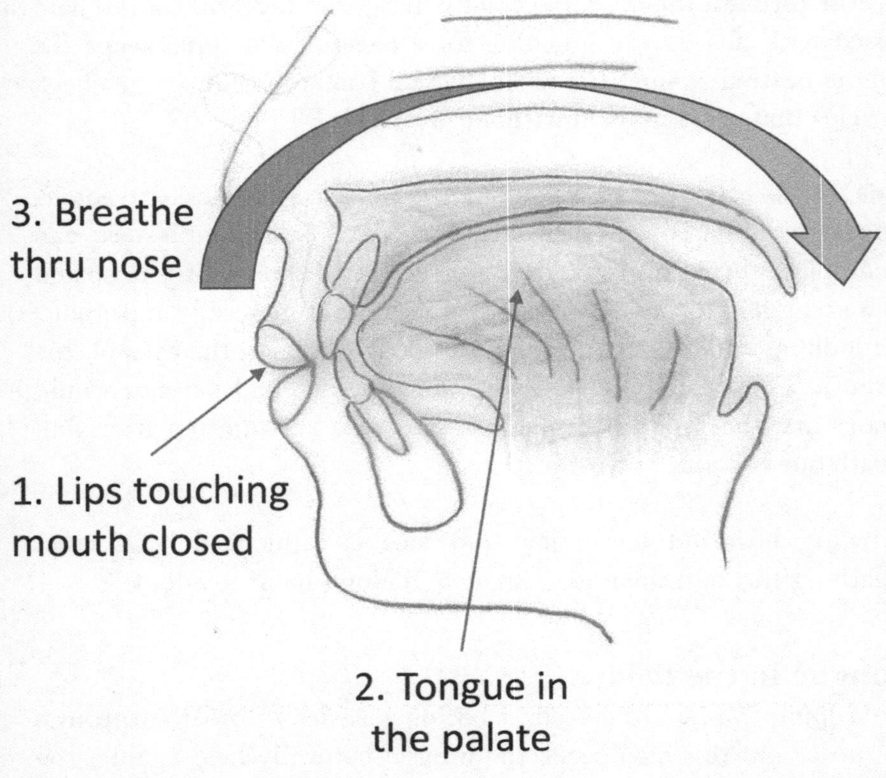
3. Breathe thru nose
1. Lips touching mouth closed
2. Tongue in the palate

Figure 11: The Big 3.

What Triggers Mouth Breathing?

We asked earlier: what may be triggering a child to breathe through an open mouth? The most obvious answer is a blocked nose and/or difficulty in breathing. Could it be an allergen or pollution in our air and environment that is causing an overreaction or hypersensitivity response leading to a congested nose?

We are observing an increased prevalence of food allergies and asthma in children in the modern world. In parallel, there seems to be a similar increase in prevalence of teeth growing crooked.

A child who finds it hard to breathe through the nose will resort to mouth breathing. As explained earlier, this results in the steepening of the palate which encroaches into the nasal cavity that lies just above. People with a deep palate and crowded teeth usually also have a deviated nasal septum and a habit of breathing through their mouth. Constant mouth opening also grows a longer and narrower face with restricted pharyngeal airway.

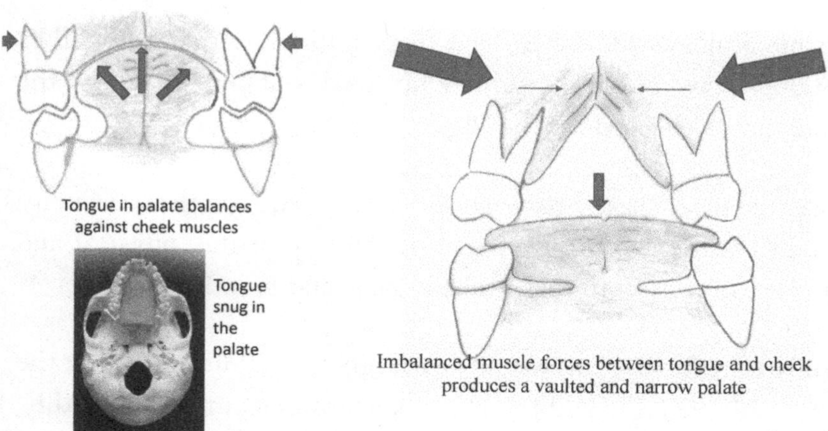

Tongue in palate balances against cheek muscles
Tongue snug in the palate
Imbalanced muscle forces between tongue and cheek produces a vaulted and narrow palate

Figure 12: Lowered tongue causes narrow palate.

Tonsils and Adenoids

Children with breathing issues and who do not breathe through the nose often have enlarged tonsils, or adenoids.

It seems to be a vicious cycle: the mouth-breathing pattern introduces unfiltered air into the throat that leads to irritation and infection of these tonsils and adenoids and, when these inflamed lymphoid tissues swell up, they further induce blockage and breathing difficulties, so the child feels the urge to continue to breathe through their mouth. Unlike inside the nose, there is no filter in the mouth to clean the inhaled air.

Parents who bring in their child to see me with dental growth concerns often add that the child also has breathing difficulties such as a blocked nose, runny nose, frequent coughs and colds. These kids may be on medications for asthma. Many of these children also have a history of having grommets or tubes placed inside their ears for improved drainage.

These medical symptoms are red flags telling us that the child's palate, upper jaw and mid face may not be developing well, and the child should be checked for the Big 3.

It is essential to see the dentist early for dentofacial growth assessment. The child's teeth and jaw have a close developmental, physical and functional connection to their ear and nose and breathing.

It is quite easy for the parents or dentist to have a quick check at the child's tonsils. Ask the child to stick their tongue out and say, 'Ahh.' The throat can be given a cursory inspection.

If parents detect or are concerned that the passage appears to be closed in, it is time to ask for a referral to an ENT doctor.

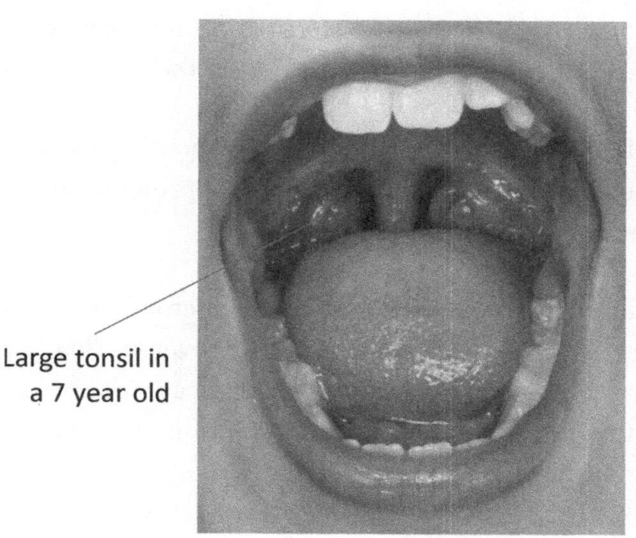

Figure 13: Large tonsils.

On that note, I add that in my experience not all ENT surgeons necessarily follow the paradigm of mouth, jaw, teeth, nose breathing, sleep and growth. Some doctors may hold the view that tonsils and adenoids will disappear with time. The doctor may only want to prescribe drugs such as antibiotics to treat the symptoms and not delve deeper into the cause of the problems or the connection with the child's disrupted sleep and dentofacial growth.

Searching for the right ENT surgeon to work with is important. Obviously, parents, physicians and dentists need to be on the same page with regards to this paradigm of health care. In recent years, I have had the good fortune of hearing many excellent paediatric sleep physicians and paediatric ENT surgeons who educate other professionals such as myself and share their views on this very interesting paradigm. They may come from different perspectives; however, not surprisingly, they all say the same thing, that nasal breathing, airway, sleep, jaw structure and tongue are related.

Breathing Retraining: The Buteyko Method

It would seem an impossible task to ask a child to not breathe through the mouth when their nose is blocked. So how can we encourage nasal breathing in this situation?

It seems like a paradox, but keeping the mouth closed will help to relieve the blocked nose. This is where the principle of the Buteyko Method of breathing retraining comes in.

Konstantin P. Buteyko was a Russian doctor and a professor in physiology. In the early 1950s, he discovered that normalizing breathing from a hyperventilating state can reverse asthma. He founded the principle that hyperventilation or over-breathing is damaging for health.[1]

The Buteyko Method trains one to not give in to the slightest urge to gasp for air, by calming and slowing down one's breathing and to always breathe only through the nose. Reducing the urge to gasp conserves the level of carbon dioxide in the lung, stops hyperventilating and effectively helps to unblock the nose.

Whilst Professor Buteyko's method originally served to treat asthma without using drugs, it turned out that the method can complement treatment for dentofacial growth by strengthening the Big 3. Dentists know that the Big 3 are essential factors for developing the maxilla and the midface, and supporting good oropharyngeal airway.

However, it is not so simple as asking a patient to just start breathing through their nose – not even for the most determined adult, let alone a young child (who has a busy mum and dad).

I see the Buteyko Method as a breathing boot camp to help break and remove bad breathing habits and effectively replace it with good, lifelong habits of calm and quiet breathing through the nose.

1. S Yakovleva, KP Buteyko & AE Novozhilov, *Breathe to Heal: Break Free from Asthma*, USA, BreathingCenter, 2016

Qualified Buteyko practitioners can be found at the Buteyko Institute of Breathing and Health (BIBH) website. I like to work with such breathing retraining specialists, allowing them to provide individual programs for my patients which will enhance their dentofacial treatment outcome.

I recommend parents to do some research and understand the amazing benefits of breathing retraining. There are many excellent online articles and useful exercises on YouTube available for free.[2,3,4,5]

Breathing retraining can ideally start from the age of about 7–8 years, and even earlier for some children. In my practice, I have observed that following a course of breathing retraining such as the Buteyko Method, the child definitely becomes more aware of how they breathe and they quite effectively change their breathing habit from using their mouth to their nose.

One is never too young or too old to learn nasal breathing. It's a matter of use it or lose it with the nose.

Forward Head Posture

Mouth breathing requires a constant open-mouth posture, and this directs lower jaw growth in a down and backward direction. A backward growing mandible further keeps the tongue closer to the throat and adds to the narrowing of the oropharynx. To compensate and regain some airway, there will be a slight head tilt-back posture at the neck.

The next compensation is by the shoulder and upper torso carrying the head down and forward to level the eyes. As the child grows, these habit and postures continue to foster growing narrower and longer faces, and also a forward head posture.

2. Dr Rosalba Courtney at https://www.rosalbacourtney.com/
3. Buteyko Clinic at https://buteykoclinic.com/
4. Buteyko Clinic YouTube channel at https://www.youtube.com/user/buteykoclinic/featured
5. Buteyko Health & Breathing (Paul O'Connell) at https://buteykoairways.com.au/

It is a common observation that forward head carriage is accompanied by a backward lower jaw and vice versa. So, a wide maxilla, forward dentofacial growth and the Big 3 equals good posture for the body.

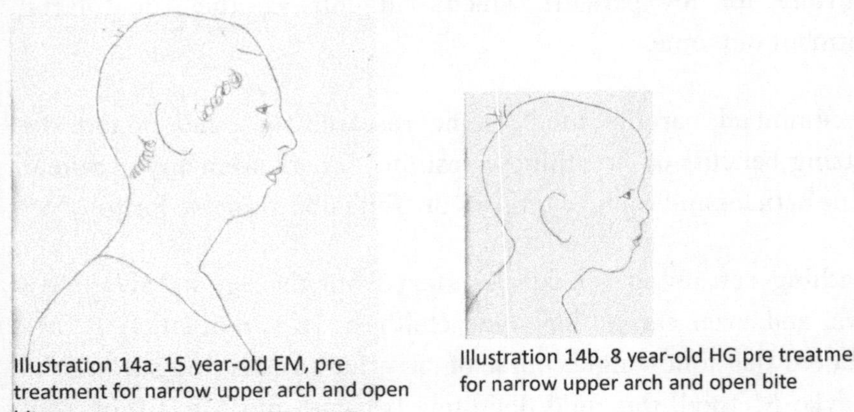

Illustration 14a. 15 year-old EM, pre treatment for narrow upper arch and open bite

Illustration 14b. 8 year-old HG pre treatment for narrow upper arch and open bite

Figure 14: Forward head posture.

Facial Beauty

Observe around you and you will see that beautiful faces with a balanced profile have the nose, lips and chin well aligned (forward). They look attractive regardless of teeth alignment.

A person with a balanced facial profile, who is breathing naturally and effortlessly through the nose will exude a universal image of good health and facial beauty regardless of their ethnicity.

By contrast, if the lower jaw and chin is not forward enough, the face will look convex and appear less attractive even if their teeth may be straight. When the midface is flat or even concave, it will detract from a beautiful face

When the upper and the lower jaws are balanced and are forward, approaching a plumb line with the nose, we see an attractive facial profile.

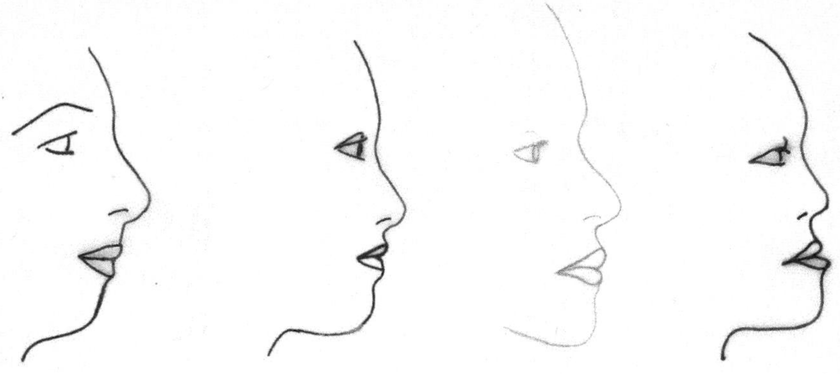

Which one do you rate as pleasing? Note that teeth do not even need to show

Figure 15: Facial profiles, convex to concave.

By contrast, when the upper and lower dental arches do not match up, a narrower upper jaw can prevent the lower jaw from relating more forward. The result can be a rather convex facial profile, with a chinless appearance as will be illustrated by the shoe diagram (see Figure 6, page 14). The nose can appear too big. We should not be blaming the nose but blaming the jaws that are too far back.

Think of nice cheek bones in a beautiful face. We do want the midface to develop forward so the lower jaw can develop forward as well to balance the upper part of the face.

Think of the nice strong jaws belonging to famous and good-looking people such as Angelina Jolie, Audrey Hepburn, Brad Pitt, Chris Hemsworth, or David Beckham and we can appreciate how the jawline enhances the perception of beauty. A forward jaw reduces the risk of the tongue blocking the airway during sleep.

We need to teach the correct habit of breathing through the nose, good tongue and jaw muscle posture and patterns through lips closure and proper chewing. This holistic and natural way to guide teeth, jaw and facial growth in the very young child will bring far reaching health rewards.

4

It's Not Just About Teeth

The modern human is susceptible to having a compromised airway that worsens when the body is in a horizontal position during sleep. When we enter the deeper stages of sleep, our muscles become totally relaxed, almost paralysed, and the throat collapses somewhat. The tongue, which is also a muscle, can become a heavy blob that falls back to block the airway, especially when one is sleeping on the back with the jaw open.

Airway blockage will compromise breathing: air intake is reduced and oxygen level in the blood drops. This is referred to as oxygen desaturation. The compromised intake of air during sleep is called sleep apnea. When the blockage is complete, the event is known as Obstructive Sleep Apnea (OSA). OSA happens not only in adults but children as well.

We also refer to this condition generally as Sleep Disordered Breathing (SDB) which explains a situation where breathing disorders take place during sleep. SDB and OSA disturb sleep and can affect the child in many serious ways such as growth, learning ability, mood, concentration, social behaviour and is linked to bruxism, and TMD and chronic pain in the older child.

So far, the reader has been alluded to the fact that there is more to it than just straight teeth. The upper and the lower jaws should be wide, and forward relative to the cranium, to give plenty of functional space for the tongue, facilitate nasal breathing, reduce the risk for compressing the TMJs, provide good airway and to enhance facial beauty.

Here are some more important factors in the equation: sleep and growth for the child.

Breathe Well to Sleep Well and to Grow Well

I want to draw the parent's attention to the fact that for your child to grow beautiful teeth, jaw and face, your child needs to sleep well. And breathing well day and night is key to their sleeping well and growing well. Correct daytime breathing through the nose may ensure that this habit is also maintained during sleep.

I often ask parents to play the role of a detective and observe how their child sleeps. Is the child able to breathe easily through the nose? Some of the clues to SDB and poor sleep include open-mouth breathing, loud snoring, laboured breathing, tossing and turning, waking during the night, nightmares and bedwetting.[6,7]

Parents will be very surprised that studies have found that there is a connection between a child's narrow palate and bedwetting during sleep.[8]

We adults know how a night of disrupted sleep or a lack of sleep can affect our state of being the following day. A child who does not sleep well is a miserable child, often with behavioural issues. In fact, more and more research studies and observations are noting the parallel symptoms of ADHD and sleep deprivation. Their learning ability and performance at school is also compromised.

---

6. DL Smith et al, Frequency of snoring, rather than apnea – hypopnea index, predicts both cognitive and behavioral problems in young children, *Sleep Medicine*, 2017 Jun; 34(2017):170-178
7. AR Jackman et al, Sleep-disordered breathing in preschool children is associated with behavioral, but not cognitive, impairments, *Sleep Medicine*, 2012;13(6):621–631.
8. U Schütz-Fransson & J Kurol, Rapid maxillary expansion effects on nocturnal enuresis in children: a follow-up study, *Angle Orthodontist*, 2008 Mar;78(2):201–8

Sleep is necessary. It is the time during the 24-hour cycle that our body rejuvenates and recharges by flushing out chemical waste in the brain. In a growing child, during the deeper phase of sleep called REM (rapid eye movement) sleep, hormones are made and released which are essential for the child's growth and development, including the formation of their brain and nervous system.

Poor quality sleep will affect the child's growth. This has become a subject of increasing concern in the health and medical arena as it should.

Posture when Sleeping

During sleep, the body is lying horizontally and since the muscles of the body become totally relaxed in the deeper phases of sleep, the tongue may fall back and further constrict the oropharynx. This may be made worse in a child with enlarged adenoids and tonsils where the blockage can become quite serious.

Airway constriction reduces the intake of air to the body, especially to the high-oxygen-consuming brain. This stresses the brain and, due to a sympathetic nervous response to the stress, the child may not be able to go into the deeper REM sleep that is essential for growth.

The child may also have disturbed sleep as the brain directs subconscious actions to gain more oxygen. The child is subconsciously aroused, stirred, unable to enter the REM phase of sleep, wakes, or even wets the bed.

When a child sleeps well, he or she will grow better, perform better and potentially make for a happier child.

Any difficulty with breathing through the nose can be made worse during the night, and the child may be forced to hang the mouth open all night. Usually, parents will also observe that the child snores and has bad breath upon rising the next morning. Whilst a mild degree of OSA is acceptable in adults, any amount of airway obstruction in a growing child has been considered unacceptable by pediatric sleep professionals.

In my practice, I routinely see worn down tooth enamel in children's teeth, and the teeth may not even be decayed. Usually, these children also have a shortened or underdeveloped upper jaw and/or they may have throats blocked by large tonsils. They tend to breathe through their mouth, not necessarily with their mouth hanging open, as sometimes this habit is not so obvious outwardly.

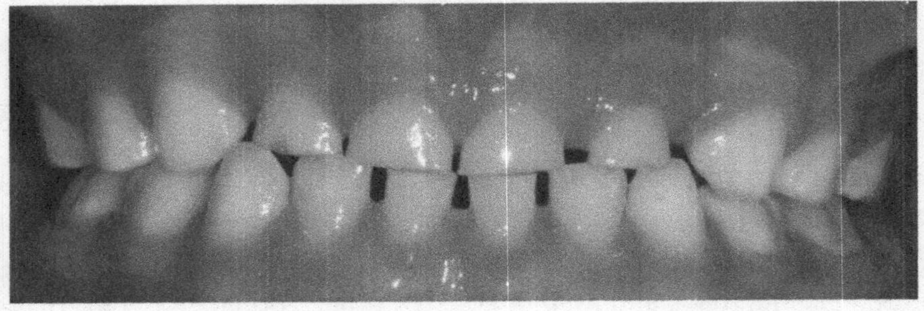

Worn teeth in a 6 year-old who bruxes during sleep. Even though there is some assuring spacing between baby teeth, this child will need sagittal maxillary development to ensure adequate room for tongue and airway, and to protect his TMJ's.

Figure 16: Six-year-old's worn front teeth.

The traditional reason given for the cause of tooth clenching and grinding is mental stress or anger. Now, contemporary observations and interpretations of tooth clenching and grinding, or **bruxing**, explain that when the airway is compromised during sleep, oxygen desaturation or oxygen deprivation triggers a sympathetic fight-or-flight response. This is big stress for the brain.

The brain is very sensitive to any fall in oxygen level in the blood and, when detected, it will cause an arousal from sleep and trigger a mouth closure or a gasp in order to reduce the throat constriction and increase air intake in an attempt to restore the oxygen level.

Bruxing brings the lower jaw closed tight against the upper jaw, and a protrusion or forward repositioning of the tongue from the throat area to improve the airflow through the throat at the back of the mouth. It is the brain's effort or attempt to remove the airway obstruction and restore oxygen level for the body.

However, the arousal or the stir from a deep sleep to restore breathing will disrupt the sleep. With chronic bruxing, the micro trauma on the TMJs can in time dislocate the jaw joints or the condyles from the disk that sits between the bony parts of the jaw joints as illustrated.

This predisposes to TMD which is more common in the child, usually an older child, than it is generally appreciated. Symptoms of TMD include TMJ pain which may also be interpreted as headaches, clicking jaw joints, limitation in jaw opening, jaw locks, and ear symptoms.

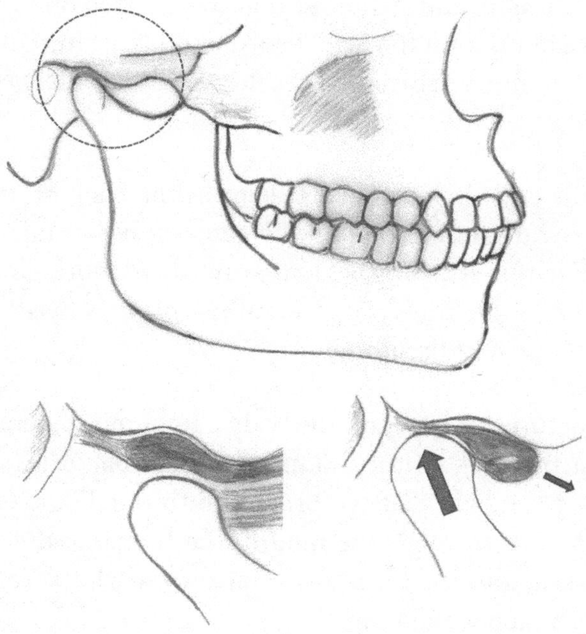

Risk for TMD when the mandible is driven back and up. The TMJ can dislocate from the disk which is pulled and trapped forward

Figure 17: Risk for TMD.

We all know how cranky we can be if we do not get a good night's sleep. There is now an appreciation of how sleep disorders can contribute to negative social behaviour in children, behaviours that parallel those observed in ADHD.[9,10,11]

As mentioned earlier, bedwetting is a symptom of sleep disorder for children. A study as far back as the 1980s had found that treating the narrow upper jaw in children stopped their bedwetting. In adults, a common symptom of OSA is the need to get up and visit the toilet during the night. Similarly, airway compromise stimulates a child to urinate in their sleep.[12]

The subject of **Tonsils and Adenoid** that we touched on in chapter 3 is revisited here in relation to sleep disordered breathing. In children one common but not exclusive cause for OSA is enlarged tonsils and/or adenoids.

Enlarged tonsils and/or adenoidal tissues at the back of the child's throat can physically block the airway causing breathing difficulty during sleep. For this reason, the dentist needs to work closely with an ENT surgeon. Sometimes, surgical intervention is needed to open the airway for improved breathing.

These soft structures are part of the body's immune system and, like gate sentries at the back of the mouth, they trap bacteria, viruses or any pollutants in the air that we breathe into our body. Obviously, when air is taken in through the mouth, the filtering effects of the nose are bypassed, and the tonsils will have to work harder to clean the air before it reaches the lungs.

Some doctors may argue that these structures will eventually shrink

9. S Moore, *Sleep-Wrecked Kids: Helping Parents Raise Happy, Healthy Kids, One Sleep at a Time*, Grammar Factory, Australia, 2018
10. JA Owens, Neurocognitive and behavioral impact of sleep disordered breathing in children, *Pediatric Pulmonology*, 2009 May; 44:417–422
11. H Andersson & L Sonnesen, Sleepiness, occlusion, dental arch and palatal dimensions in children attention deficit hyperactivity disorder (ADHD), *European Archives of Paediatric Dentistry*, 2018 Apr;19(2):91–97
12. M Zaffanello et al, Obstructive sleep-disordered breathing, enuresis and combined disorders in children: chance or related association?, *Swiss Medical Weekly*, 2017 Feb;147:w14400

away and therefore advocate against its removal. However, according to the British Lung Foundation there is good reason to have these obstructive structures removed during this important growing stage for the child.[13]

Parents will have to weigh up the benefits gained by solving the immediate problem of apnea and nightly sleep deprivation, against the negative impact of a surgery under general anesthesia.

Encouraging the child to sleep with a closed mouth and to breathe through the nose will ensure that air is cleaned and filtered at the entrance. This is obviously nature's preferred way. The tonsillar tissues will then not have to deal with an overload situation.

13. BritLungFoundation, 2013 Feb 12, *The effects of OSA*, video, viewed 2018 Sep, https://www.youtube.com/watch?v=UuvsYf12Gb8

5

When to Start?

To avoid having crowded and crooked teeth in adulthood, the child's jaws need to grow wide and forward to provide room for permanent teeth, which are much larger than the deciduous or milk teeth. Jaw growth is a process that begins from birth and parents have a significant role in stimulating this growth.

We have discussed how the earlier we keep a lookout and keep steering growth on the right track, the better. The younger the child, the easier it is, as their skeleton is more adaptable. Many ancient cultures have exploited this flexibility; for example, Chinese foot-binding, Burmese neck elongation and South American skull elongation. For the jaws, breastfeeding is the first action in the stimulation for growth, well before any tooth erupts in the mouth.

Importance of Breastfeeding

The newborn has no teeth; however, nature is so clever to design breastfeeding not just as a way for the baby to get fed with the right nutrients, but also as a stimulus for good dental development.

Instinctively, the baby's mouth closes neatly over the mother's breast nipple to form a seal, whilst the forward part of the tongue cups under the nipple, and the back part moves up and down against the palate to create a vacuum in the mouth that draws the milk from the breast. The baby then holds the milk momentarily before swallowing, following a rhythmic sequence of suckle-swallow-breathe (through the nose).

This rhythmic pumping of the baby's lower jaw, and pressing of the nipple by the tongue against the palate stimulates the jaws and the midface structure to grow. The mother's nipple is the perfect mould for the baby's mouth whilst the jaw, tongue and mouth muscles make the perfect pump.

Feeding posture: The aim is to facilitate a good oral seal by the baby's lips and tongue around the breast to prevent air leakage and intake, and to enable nasal breathing. With breastfeeding the baby can be held more upright, keeping its neck and body straight and overextension of the neck is prevented. The nose should be next to the breast. Holding the baby more upright prevents milk from flowing back up towards the oesophagus resulting in a reflux. Keeping the ear above mouth level prevents backflow of milk into the ear that may cause ear infection.

Just the right feeding amount: Overfeeding can lead to reflux or regurgitation of milk from the baby's stomach. Studies have found that babies need very little milk, about the size of its fist, at any one time. This may be reassuring for some mothers who are concerned that they do not have enough milk for the baby. If the milk flows too fast, then it can cause stress for the baby in keeping up the feed-swallow-breathe rhythm. Breastfeeding gives the baby a better control of rate of milk flow.

In my practice, I have observed that despite the baby having been breastfed, there may still be issues with underdeveloped jaws and/or tooth crowding as the child's teeth begin to appear. This is because there are always many layers of environmental and genetic influence on jaw and teeth growth. Nonetheless, breastfeeding is still an early insurance for the maxilla to grow unhindered. It will help reduce any negative impact so that even if there may be a need for a correction of any shortcoming, the corrective measures will be easier.

Growth and development of the jaw-face-teeth complex is not so much an evolutionary change that requires many generations, but rather it is an adaptation influenced by the functioning of the tongue and cheek muscles which commences early in infancy.

Mother's Health during Pregnancy

Before birth, it is important for the pregnant mother to maintain good health to pass on the benefits as well as reduce any unwanted stress to the foetus, particularly by:

- breathing well through the nose
- ensuring adequate restorative REM sleep
- paying attention to diet and ensuring adequate nutrition
- reducing any risk of high blood pressure
- reducing any need for taking medication, especially antibiotics.
- avoiding alcohol

Towards the third trimester of pregnancy, there is an increased risk for a temporary development of OSA for the mother. This condition can lead to oxygen desaturation, arousal and disturbances and high blood pressure during sleep which should be assessed and treated by the family doctor and with a referral to a sleep physician as necessary.[14,15]

Some treatment with medication for the mother has been linked to the development of various tooth enamel defects for the child. These defects can be visible on front teeth and unsightly. Tooth enamel defects can occur during the early stages of tooth formation. The child's baby teeth are affected by factors occurring from the second trimester of pregnancy, whilst permanent or adult tooth defects can arise from factors occurring at or soon after birth, and up to five years of age.

---

14. J Dominguez et al, Recognition of obstructive sleep apnea in pregnancy survey, *International Journal of Obstetric Anaesthesia*, 2016; 26: 85–7.
15. LM O'Brien et al, Hypertension, Snoring, and Obstructive Sleep Apnea During Pregnancy: A Cohort Study, *BJOG*, 2014 Dec; 121(13): 1685–1693.

Breast Milk: Some mothers pump their breast milk and store it in bottles so their baby can feed on demand when the mother may have to go to work.

Remember that this is more than about the contents of the milk. It is also about the baby suckling the mother's nipple to express the breast milk. It is about the baby's tongue and the breast nipple fitting snugly against the baby's palate in order to stimulate the development of the palate, and ultimately the dentofacial structure, to its full potential.

Is Bottle Feeding Good Enough?

Mothers who bottle feed their babies would need to keep in mind the importance of the position and posture of the baby during feeding, the rate of flow from the holes made in the teat, the shape, length and firmness of the teat for an effective suckle by the baby. Also check the nutritive content of the non-human milk formulae and the freshness of the milk stored in the bottle.

The baby breathes and swallows more easily when breastfeeding because the milk flow from the breast is controlled by the baby's suckling and not by gravity as with bottle feeding. The consensus is that it is not possible to find a milk bottle and teat that can be as effective as a human nipple and breast.

The rhythmic pressing of the lower jaw and tongue and mother's nipple against the palate and the contraction of the cheek muscles create the stimulus for the growth of the palate. A flat palate does not encroach into the nose cavity or impairs airway that is so important for proper nasal breathing.

Generally, it is recommended that a newborn be breastfed exclusively for at least 6 months and partially up to 12 months or much longer for good dentofacial growth and general good health for the baby.

In Asia, where I was born and brought up, it was not uncommon for a family to hire a 'wet nurse' to feed the baby should the mother not be able to breastfeed the child for any reason such as illness. This would have been the normal child care practice in the past before bottles, teats and baby formula were invented.

Observations have been made that in cultures where breastfeeding is the normal and only available practice, and especially if the community live entirely on natural and non-processed food, the child tends to grow beautiful wide jaws that can accommodate all 32 adult teeth, including the wisdom teeth. Tooth crowding is rare, in contrast to what we see in our modern culture.

Mothers' milk is also the perfect formula for the infant that no commercial product can substitute. This milk is free, is always freshly made, and provides all the nutrients, proteins, fat, carbs, vitamins and even antibodies the child needs without any risk of malnutrition and/or allergy to a non-human formula 'milk'. However, I qualify here that the mother needs to ensure that she is on a balanced diet that provides all the minerals and nutrients she needs for herself and to pass on to the baby via her milk.

WHO's concern: On the Australian ABC Radio midday news in October 2017, it was reported that Australian mothers of newborns are lagging behind in breastfeeding. The international rate for breastfeeding is 40%, whilst in Australia only 10 to 15% of mothers breastfeed their baby up to 6 months.

This report was given by Dr Howard Sobel, head of Child Health and Nutrition. He is also the south-eastern regional representative of the World Health Organisation (WHO). He said, 'Babies who are not breastfed entirely are 10 times more likely to be sick and to die, at least in poorer countries. Fast feed infant formulae may be equated to junk food with all its artificial contents.'

Breastfeeding can reduce chronic diseases: A research done by ANU's Australian Centre for Economic Research on Health, published in 2010 in the International Journal of Public Health Nutrition had found that breastfeeding can reduce the risk of chronic diseases.[16]

---

16. JP Smith & PJ Harvey PJ, Chronic disease and infant nutrition: is it significant to public health?, *Cambridge University Press*, 2011;14(2):279–89.

The study was set out to assess the public health significance of premature weaning of infants from breast milk on the risk of chronic illnesses in later life. The study mapped the public health impact of premature weaning from breastfeeding over a period of five decades in Australia. The research showed that negative attitudes to breastfeeding may have contributed to a rise in chronic disease in Australia especially among disadvantaged families.

During the 1960s, 90% of people were weaned off breastfeeding before they were six months old due to unsupportive health policies and negative public attitude in the post-war years. These people would now be in their 40s and 50s. The researchers suggested that from what they know about the effects of premature weaning, a significant proportion of the current burden of chronic disease might have been avoided had they been breastfed longer.

They also suggested more should be done to promote breastfeeding past the age of six months to mitigate the risk of chronic disease in the future. The researchers found that there are few preventative health interventions like breastfeeding that shows consistent, long-term effects in reducing chronic disease.

As previously mentioned, in communities where breastfeeding is the only way, the child has well-developed dental arches. Other dentists and medical professionals have made similar observations and wrote about their concerns with the current trend away from breastfeeding, albeit from slightly different approaches.[17,18]

In summary, the benefits of breastfeeding for a child include nutritional, immunological, emotional, psychological and the practice is also foundational to dentofacial growth.

Pure breastfeeding for at least six months is positively associated with good dental arch development that will give a reduced chance of developing dental malocclusion.

17. BG Palmer, 2003 Mar 4, *The Uniqueness of the Human Airway*, Sleep Review, viewed 2018 Sep, http://www.sleepreviewmag.com/2003/03/the-uniqueness-of-the-human-airway/
18. SY Park, *Sleep, Interrupted*, Jodev Press, USA, 2012, p.17

Could it be that in our modern civilisation, where breastfeeding is no longer the only option and is less popular, that we are seeing a concomitant rise in the prevalence of crooked teeth?

Mothers are encouraged not to give in to formula and bottle feeding too readily.

Tongue-tie

Tongue-tie is an important topic relating to breastfeeding, dentofacial growth and development, and other significant health issues. A tied tongue, or tongue-tie, is often heard of but its significance seemingly poorly understood.[19]

The medical term is 'ankyloglossia' and in more recent times it is also referred to as 'tethered oral tissues' or TOT. It refers to the abnormally tight oral tissue attachment under the tongue that anchors or tethers the tongue to the floor of the mouth, limiting the movement of the tongue. There are varying degrees of tongue-tie and movement limitations. There are also 'lip-ties' that tether the upper or lower lip to the respective gum area of the jaw. Tongue-ties are common.

Whenever there is any issue with breastfeeding, such as pain experienced by the mother and/or an inability for the baby to latch on for an effective feed, the underside of the tongue should be inspected for any tight restriction by running a finger under the tongue, then all around to detect any restriction to the finger movement.

A tethered tongue can cause the baby to struggle to stretch its tongue forward to cup under the nipple. This can render the mouth seal ineffective, and the baby ends up sucking in and swallowing air. Aerophagia can cause distension of the baby's tummy, discomfort and pain, and reflux.

19. DMB Hall & MJ Renfrew, Tongue tie, *Archives of Disease in Childhood*, 2005 Nov;90;1211–1215

Tongue-tie can also cause pain for the mother as the baby struggles and compensates with its jaw or emerging teeth for an effective latch. This is one reason for many mums to give up breastfeeding. In fact, tongue-tie can also affect and cause frustration for the mum and baby equally with bottle feeding.

Other clues to this restrictive tether include the heart-shaped appearance of the tongue when the baby cries and has its mouth open, or an obvious firm attachment of the tongue tip by the tie, or the appearance of a white coating of milk residue on the back of the tongue indicating an ineffective swallow due to the restriction.

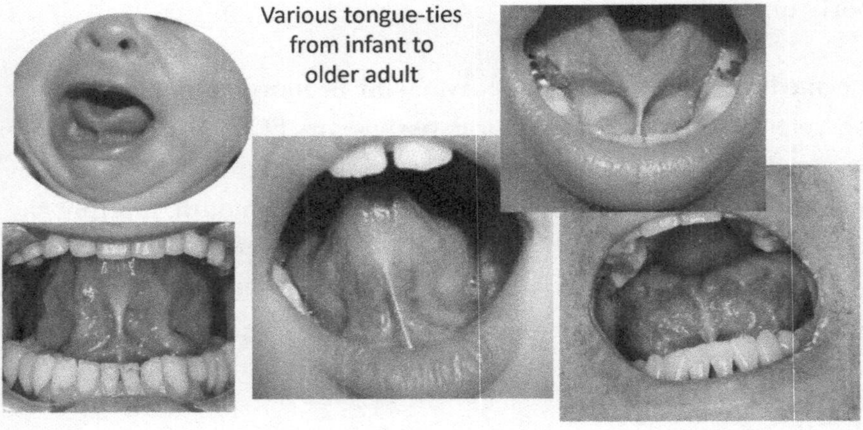

Various tongue-ties
from infant to
older adult

Figure 18: Tongue-ties.

Tongue-tie release: When I was a dental student, I learnt surgical techniques to release a tied-tongue, but we were taught to do this only in an older child or adult with a speech impediment. There was no concern for the fact that a tied-tongue prevents a newborn from suckling the mother's breast effectively nor that this should be assessed for an early release.

Surgical techniques for releasing a tied tongue include the use of surgical scissors, scalpels or laser knife (also known as ablation). Normally, this is released under some local analgesia. The younger the baby, the easier to treat and with less disruption.

In fact, the release is even performed without local analgesia in the newborn. It is a simple procedure with no report of adverse events. Immediately following the release, the baby can return to the mum's breast, to be comforted by the improved ease of suckling.

In an older child, local analgesia will be required, and scarring may be a side effect. Also, pre- and post-surgery stretching exercises are required for a good outcome.

The tissue that ties the tongue to the floor of the mouth is known as the frenum or frenulum. And the surgical release and removal of a tight frenulum is therefore referred to as a 'frenulectomy' or abbreviated to 'frenectomy'. A most simple procedure that does not involve any removal of tissue at all is also called a 'frenotomy'. Other terms used for procedures for releasing a tied-tongue are revision or division of the tongue.

If left untreated, tongue-ties can encourage a disconnect between the tongue and the palate, lead to orofacial myology disorders and therefore affect dentofacial growth and development. Other ramifications may include speech and eating impediments, negative behavioural and social impact. It has now been observed that tongue-tie is linked to airway problems, specifically OSA in children.[20]

The significance and importance of tied-tongues are so much appreciated in **Brazil** that they passed a national health regulation in 2004 requiring that every newborn's frenulum be inspected and, if necessary, be released for improved breastfeeding and the benefit of proper dentofacial growth and development of an optimal airway.

I heard that in ancient times, immediately following birth the midwife would routinely check under the newborn's tongue for any tongue-tie and she would not hesitate to nick a tethered tongue using her fingernail if necessary. It does seem barbaric to us but perhaps these ancient people were wiser than we care to appreciate, and they would have been successful for thousands of years practising what was good for the baby.

---

20. C Guilleminault, S Huseni & L Lo, A frequent phenotype for paediatric sleep apnoea: short lingual frenulum, *ERJ Open Research*, 2016 Feb:00043-2016

Lip-ties: It is common to see a smile showing a gap between the middle permanent upper-front teeth. These teeth are separated by a thick band of oral tissue which also ties the upper lip to the upper jaw bone and can restrict the movement of the lip.

Similar to a tongue-tie, a lip-tie in the newborn can interfere with effective breastfeeding, though according to some doctors who treat these conditions, a lip-tie may be secondary to the tongue-tie. So, look out for tongue-ties first.

As teeth erupt into the mouth, a lip-tie can interfere with proper oral muscular function, preventing teeth from being effectively swiped clean by the tongue and lips and thus causing tooth decay. Therefore, children should be inspected for this restriction and have the lip-tie released as necessary. I recommend the book *SOS 4 TOTS* by Dr Lawrence A. Kotlow to learn more details about these tissue tethers.

Adults with tongue-ties: In my dental practice nowadays, I look out for tongue-ties in all my patients. I see a great number of adults (approximately 60%) with varying degrees of tether. Releasing a tongue-tie was obviously not the trend when these adults were born. I observe that most of these adults also have underdeveloped jaws, sleep-disordered breathing, TMD and poor dental occlusion.

Of course, a frenulectomy can be done at any age and adults who have had this done are known to report a sense of release in their upper body girdle, ease of stretching, improved breathing and sleeping, and/or reduction of chronic pain.

Real Food for Great Teeth

When the infant transitions from breastfeeding to eating solid food as teeth begin to erupt, the child should be given real food with good nutritional value and food with various textures to learn to chew.

There is an increasing awareness of the harmful effects of sugar on not just teeth but also on general health. (Anyone who has not yet seen it should see That Sugar Film.) Beware that there is much hidden sugar in processed and packaged food that is commonly touted as healthy. These include cereals, fruit juices and low-fat dairy products. Some food can be allergenic and may cause nose congestions and blockages.

Parents should take the opportunity whilst the child is very young and still under the parents' control to get them used to eating real, natural foods that does not come out of a packet or a tube. There are many dietary guidelines on the internet and since I am not a dietitian, I am not able to be giving detailed advice on what your family should be eating. Parents should make educated decisions for the child on what to eat and set examples of good eating habits and food choices.

Nevertheless, I generally recommend:

- to not add sugar to your child's food and drinks
- that consumption of foods containing sugar should be minimised and your child must learn that this type of food is not for daily consumption
- to train your child to enjoy food that is natural and to consistently develop such a healthy habit
- to have your child learn that water is a great drink on its own
- that your child needs sufficient amounts of fat-soluble vitamins such as vitamin D, A and K2 to aid absorption of calcium for the growth of teeth and bones
- to read Dr Steven Lin's book called *The Dental Diet* for a more comprehensive dietary guideline.

It is important to note though that jaw muscle development, like many other areas of the body, relies on good exercises. So, the more chewing of fibrous or sinewy foods, such as raw fruit, vegetables and meat, the better.

Baby food may be cooked soft especially for when the teeth are just starting to come through but, as soon as possible, give a piece of lamb chop or chicken drumstick for the child to hold and to gnaw.

A piece of raw carrot or any piece of vegetable which is crunchy or chewy may also be suitable.

These are foods that our hunter-gatherer ancestors gave to their children and, according to findings, they had wide, strong jaws with plenty of room for all their teeth. Real and natural food is best.

Thumb or Dummy Sucking

Discourage thumb or finger sucking habits from a young age. These harmful habits tend to stay with the child for far too long and can be challenging to get rid of.

When teeth begin to come through, any such lingering finger or thumb-sucking habits can cause distortion in tooth alignment, resulting in an open bite or the bucked teeth appearance. Thumb sucking can distort the maxilla, forming an exaggerated narrow V-shape. It can drive the mandible back distally. And it obviously works against the Big 3 principle.

There is an explanation offered that a child wants to suck their thumb or finger because it provides comfort from the contact with the palate. An alternate view is that the child does this as a need to swallow to suppress an urge to reflux.

Whatever may be triggering these habits, they should be promptly discouraged. There are healthier ways to replace these sucking habits. Of course, the child should be using the tongue instead. The earlier we start on any such habit correction, the easier it will be.

Apart from OM Therapy (see Chapter 7), there are some helpful tools to use under the guidance of the parents and dentist. For example, Myo Munchee (https://myomunchee.com) is a great little oral device that is particularly suitable for young children from 2–5 years old. When worn, it helps stimulates salivary flow, cleans teeth, trains to keep the mouth closed and to exercise lips and jaw muscles – all necessary for optimal dentofacial growth.

Myobrace (https://myobrace.com) is another excellent product line which is designed to help the child achieve the Big 3.

If possible, do not replace the thumb with a dummy (also known as pacifier in some countries) although, admittedly, the dummy may be easier to get rid of than the thumb or finger. It can also cause an open bite, distorts tooth alignment and works against the Big 3 principle.

Preventing Early Loss

Early loss of baby teeth, especially back teeth, may allow neighbouring teeth to creep into the empty space that is left, which can result in crowding and crookedness when adult teeth later attempt to erupt into the assigned space. This can be prevented by good oral hygiene which should be taught to children as early as possible. Parents should set a good example. Flossing between your child's back teeth (deciduous molars) can and should be carried out by parents regularly.

Summary

- Breastfeed for at least 6 months, ideally 12 months or even longer.
- Feeding with a bottle is not quite the same. The artificial teat does not have the same structure as a mother's breast nipple. It is not just about getting the best nutrients from the mother's milk, it is also about the suckling as a stimulation for palate growth.
- Tongue tether? Ensure baby's tongue can move freely to enable a good latch onto mother's nipple.
- Transition to real, unprocessed food with various textures for the baby to learn to eat properly. No mushy food from a tube. Teach the baby to eat with mouth closed and to chew properly.
- Observe and encourage the Big 3.
- Teach baby to always breathe through the nose, but make sure nose is not easily blocked. Check tonsils and avoid any food that may promote excessive production of mucus.
- Avoid or be prepared to terminate the need to use a dummy or pacifier early.
- Prevent early loss of baby teeth: maintain good dental hygiene and low exposure to sugar.

6

The Clues to Look for in Your Child

In the previous chapters, I advised parents to take simple steps **early** to give their child the best chance to grow gorgeous teeth, beautiful jaw and face, and have broad, winning smiles. Keeping an eye on this important area of growth that is usually referred to as dentofacial growth must continue throughout the child's early years, especially in the first 6–8 years of their life.

When growth is not tracking right, redirection will be easier when the child is young and their structure is amazingly adaptable. The child will also have fewer outside social influences to deal with at that time of life.

A child's growth in the cranium and jaw is already 80% complete by the time they are 8 years of age, or even earlier in girls. Because of this, the clues also present themselves early. By being aware of them, you will be able to take steps early and intercept an undesirable growth trend that could lead to bigger and more costly issues in the future.

As a general dentist, I also treat adults in my practice and I can confirm that these growth problems, if left untreated, will not solve themselves as the child transitions into adulthood. Just as we are observing an increase of a need for tooth straightening, there is also an all-time high prevalence of chronic pain associated with the jaw, head and neck as well as a high prevalence of obstructive sleep apnoea (OSA) or breathing related sleep issues seen in the adult population.

Parents will save money and heartache by mitigating complicated treatments that can become necessary if growth problem is allowed to develop unchecked.

The clues to look out for are:

- undersized upper jaw and abnormal bites
- functional issues
    - » poor oral muscle habits and posture
    - » poor breathing patterns
    - » nose, throat and ear issues
- unsatisfactory facial profile
- If parent(s) of the child have any of the above conditions and/or SDB.

These issues often do not occur in isolation but can be present together to varying degrees because, in some way, they are all linked to inadequate maxilla growth. I highlight the more common clues below.

Children with the dreaded Bucky Beaver look (**buckteeth**) are prone to injuring their upper-front teeth. While it seems logical to blame the upper teeth that appear to be sticking out, it is in fact more common that the mandible is trapped too far back because the upper dental arch is too tapered. Beware of any treatment that aims at retracting the upper-front teeth back to match up with the ill-positioned mandible (see Figures 6 and 8 in Chapter 2).

Often, the lower lip will get caught in the large space behind the erupting upper incisors, thus perpetuating the large overjet.

Crowding is a red flag for an undersized jaw. One of the most common concerns for parents is to notice a new, permanent lower-front tooth (incisor) erupting behind the baby teeth crowded out of alignment.

Crowding of lower incisors when the maxilla is not large enough...

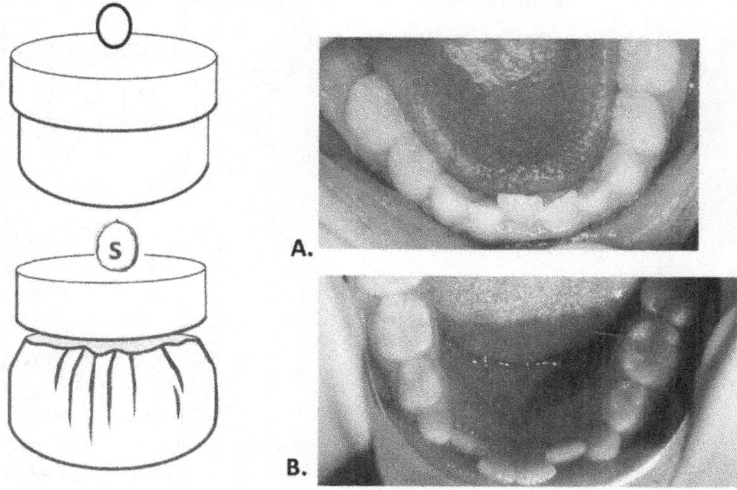

Figure 19: Crowding.

Other common areas for crowding include the upper incisors and canines as these adult teeth begin to come through.

Overbite, underbite, deep bite and crossbite: in primary dentition, the upper-front teeth normally overlap or cover the outside of the lower-front teeth by about 20–30% of the height of the lower incisors. This is called a (normal) **overbite**. As they transition to adult dentition, the front teeth overbite should reduce to approximately 10–15% of the height of the lower incisors. (See Figure 5 in Chapter 2.)

Too much overbite (greater than 30%) is referred to as a deep overbite, or simply **deep bite**. Too little or no overbite would indicate an undersized upper jaw. The upper teeth should not meet edge on with the lower teeth.

The analogy is a hat box that should have a lid (the upper dental arch) that is slightly larger to cover the box (lower dental arch). If the lid is too small, then the two parts will not fit together properly.

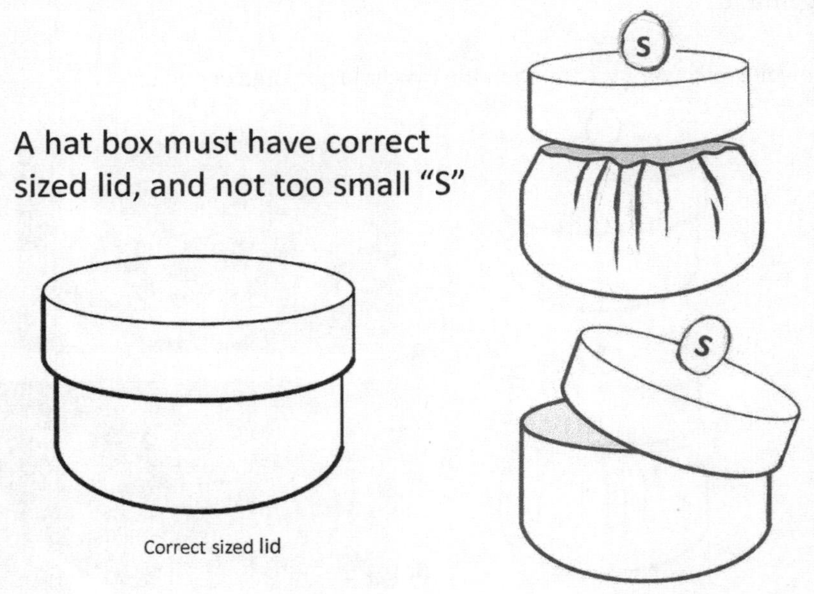
A hat box must have correct sized lid, and not too small "S"
S
S
Correct sized lid

Figure 20: Hat box and lids.

A **crossbite** results when the overlap is reversed; that is, the upper teeth fit inside to the lower teeth. The cause is a disproportion in jaw sizes, with the upper being relatively undersized.

The crossbite may be located between the front teeth. The lay term for this is an **underbite.** This often presents in a child who has a genetic predisposition to a strong lower jaw growth.

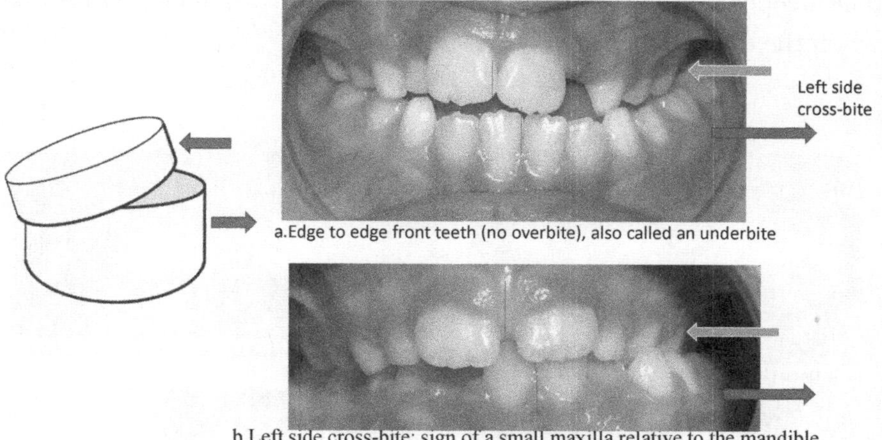

Left side
cross-bite
a.Edge to edge front teeth (no overbite), also called an underbite
b.Left side cross-bite: sign of a small maxilla relative to the mandible

Figure 21: Left side crossbite.

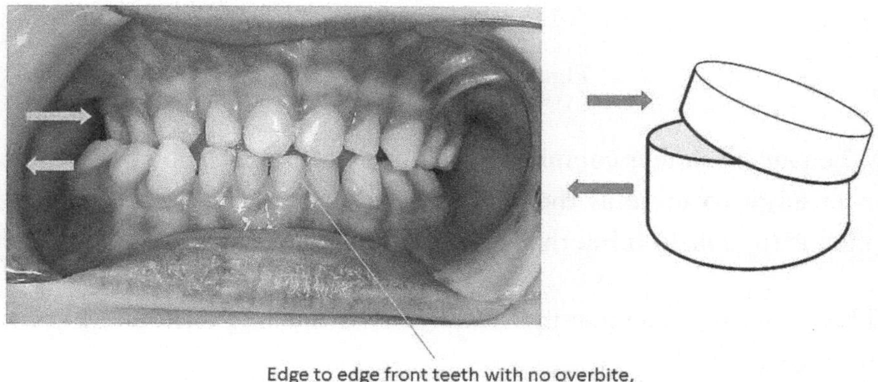

Edge to edge front teeth with no overbite,
common sign of a under-sized maxilla,
relative to the mandible

Figure 22: Right side crossbite.

A subtle indication of an underbite is when the upper incisors do not show as much as the lower-front teeth when smiling. Normally, when smiling, the upper incisors should show more than the lower.

A **deep bite** is when the upper teeth overlap the lower teeth by more than 30%.

The deeper the overbite, the less the lower-front teeth will show when the child close the teeth together.

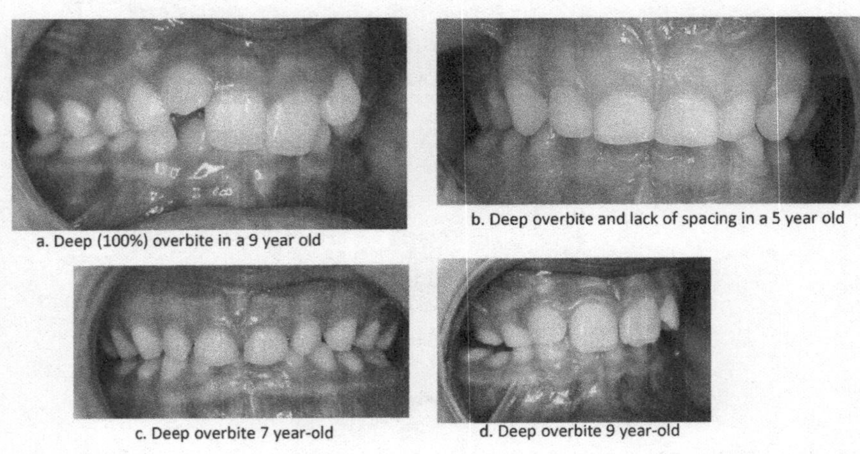

a. Deep (100%) overbite in a 9 year old

b. Deep overbite and lack of spacing in a 5 year old

c. Deep overbite 7 year-old

d. Deep overbite 9 year-old

Figure 23: Deep overbite.

When an overbite is completely lacking – that is, the baby front teeth meet **edge to edge** as the child closes the jaws together – parents often erroneously think this is how it should be.

This is an early clue that upper jaw growth is insufficient (see Figure 16 in Chapter 4).

In a **gummy smile**, there is excessive display of the pink gums above the upper-front teeth, as if the whole upper dental arch has grown too far down. This can be seen even in the very young and is common for adults as well.

Growth in a downward direction moves the lower jaw and tongue further back and predisposes the child to having a restricted airway and TMD.

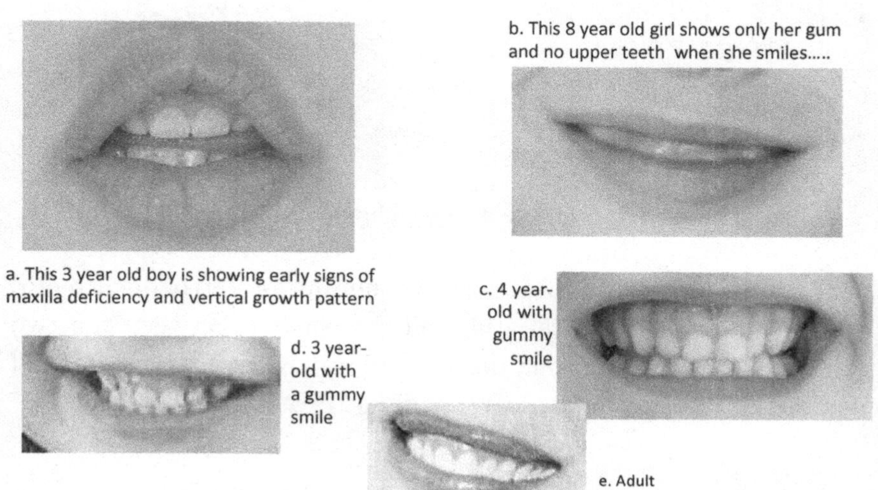

b. This 8 year old girl shows only her gum and no upper teeth when she smiles.....
a. This 3 year old boy is showing early signs of maxilla deficiency and vertical growth pattern
c. 4 year-old with gummy smile
d. 3 year-old with a gummy smile
e. Adult

Figure 24: Gummy smiles – excessive gum display in the upper arch.

An **open bite** is usually the result of a prolonged sucking of the dummy or the child's thumb or finger. Prolonged placement of these items between the front teeth prevent the teeth from coupling or to close together.

This is a problem worth treating early.

An open bite can also be the result of a severe open-mouth breathing habit and poor oral muscle patterns that allow the tongue to constantly sit between the incisors. Prevent an open bite by encouraging mouth closure at a young age.

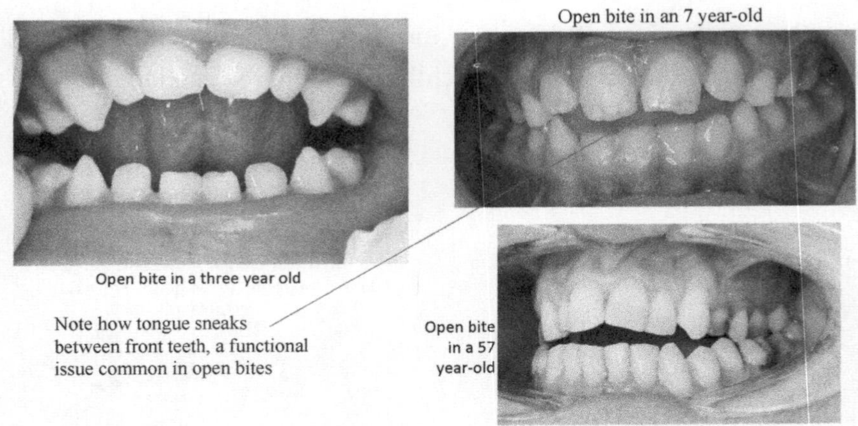

Open bite in an 7 year-old
Open bite in a three year old
Note how tongue sneaks between front teeth, a functional issue common in open bites
Open bite in a 57 year-old

Figure 25: Open bites.

Teeth leaning inwards (inadequate proclining or retroclined teeth) forms an undersized dental arch and a mismatch between the two arches will result. This may be evident in the primary teeth and when the adult upper incisors are coming through.

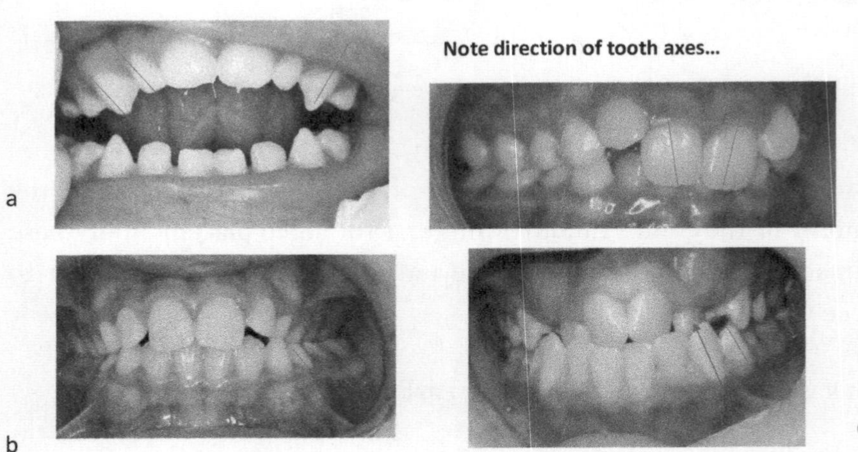

Note direction of tooth axes...

Retroclined teeth (leaning inwards) in primary and adult dentition. Smaller dental arches result.

Figure 26: Retroclined teeth.

The less obvious clue to an undersized palate or upper jaw is the **lack of spacings** between the child's primary teeth. From about the age of 4 years, the jaw should enlarge to prepare for the arrival of the second set of larger teeth and, during the transition, the smaller baby teeth will appear too tiny for the growing jaw with the front baby teeth showing some spacings between them. If spacing is not obvious, then this is an early warning that the upper jaw may not be growing to its maximum potential.

It may be difficult for the parents to know just how much spacing is considered to be normal between the child's growing teeth. Your family dentist should be able to monitor and advise you in this regard.[21]

Just a word of caution here: if there is a bad tongue habit where the tongue thrusts forward constantly pushing against the upper-front teeth, this can splay or spread the front teeth apart resulting in larger gaps. This is not normal either.

Usually, in this instance, the upper-front teeth will assume a jutting forward appearance. This undesirable tongue habit is also known as an **infantile swallow** or a **tongue-thrust** habit.

Other **poor muscle habit red flags** include excessive drooling, mouth-breathing, mouth hanging open constantly, dried flaky lips or swollen and reddish lips (especially the lower), messy eating with food spilling out of the mouth, and difficulty in swallowing food (with tongue thrusting out).

A child should be trained to chew their food with their mouth closed and with no talking. Parents should enforce this habit by setting a good example in doing the same.

Parents and dentist may need to work closely with a dedicated orofacial myotherapist to retrain the use of these mouth muscles.

---

21. Helpful reference for dental growth chart: https://www.pinterest.co.uk/pin/503699539556188735/?lp=true

Parents often report to me that they can hear their child **grind teeth loudly** during the night. The child will have flattened and **worn teeth**, with significant loss of tooth enamel.

An underdeveloped upper jaw presents an increased risk for airway restriction, which is usually worse during sleep. The child may have some degree of SDB or apnea which in turn predisposes the child to tooth clenching and grinding. (Refer to chapter 4 for more details.)

Edge-to-edge front teeth and bruxing during sleep are red flags for SDB which should alert the parents to seek early intervention to help the upper jaw grow more. Seek help from your dentist to manage this issue early (see Figure 16 in Chapter 4). Does your child experience **breathing difficulties**? Look out for where the mouth stays open all the time or if there is a constant **blocked nose**.

Snoring during sleep should be investigated to rule out any SDB. Clues to disturbed sleep include **daytime tiredness** and excessive **yawning**, and social behaviour parallel to those in children with ADHD.[22,23]

---

22. JA Owens, Neurocognitive and behavioral impact of sleep disordered breathing in children, *Pediatric Pulmonology*, 2009 May; 44:417–422
23. H Andersson & L Sonnesen, Sleepiness, occlusion, dental arch and palatal dimensions in children attention deficit hyperactivity disorder (ADHD), *European Archives of Paediatric Dentistry*, 2018 Apr;19(2):91–97

Adenoid face refers to a facial appearance displaying a narrow and long face usually associated with an open-mouth breathing habit due to chronic nasal blockages and enlarged adenoids which prevents the child from breathing through the nose.

The midface or cheeks are flat with poor muscle tone. Because of the insufficient midface structure, venous circulation is affected, and so these kids tend to have dark or bluey shadows below the eyes (known as venous pooling). The constant open-mouth habit affects the jaw muscles such that the child tends to have a convex facial profile with a receded chin.

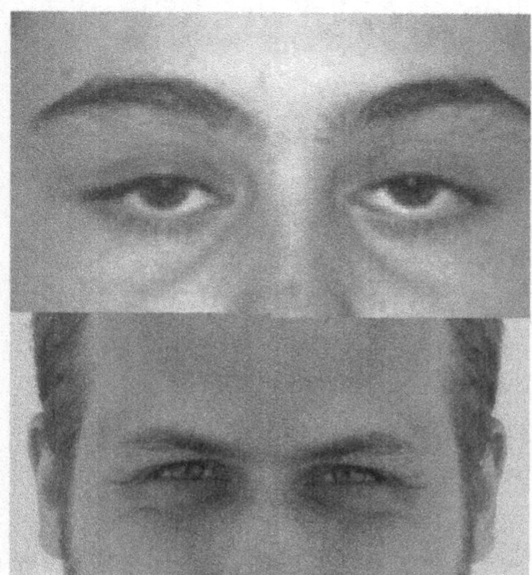

Characteristics of an adenoid face:

Poor maxilla development- jaws set back
Poor vein drainage = venous pooling, shadow below eyes
Tired droopy eyes, white below iris showing
Flat cheeks, bags below eyes
Blocked nose, snuffy, rhinitis
Mouth-breathing
Long and narrow face

Figure 27: Adenoid face.

Shape and size of teeth. A question I often get asked is that can the jaw be too small and the teeth too large? This is a widely held belief and perhaps an excuse given for removal of teeth that are blamed to be taking up too much space. The reality is that the incidence of such freakish disproportion is extremely rare in nature. My motto is to develop the jaw first before considering if it is necessary to remove healthy teeth.

By contrast, the permanent teeth can sometimes turn out to be too small (the technical term is 'microdontia') and this is commonly presented as a pair of very narrow or **peg-shaped upper lateral incisors**. For good looks, these teeth will need to be cosmetically built out (we do this later in adulthood) so that the size of these skinny teeth will be proportional and harmonious with the other permanent incisors. Such a balance will improve the smile and fit in with our goal for optimally wide dental arches that can satisfactorily accommodate the tongue.

Beware that these disproportionally skinny lateral incisors do not take up as much space and therefore parents can be lulled into a false sense of security thinking that all is fine when they do not see any evidence of crowding. Even though these narrow teeth may need less dental arch space, the child still needs a well-developed palate and wide dental arches to accommodate the tongue!

The extreme of such narrow teeth would be a lack of these teeth altogether, a condition known as 'dental agenesis' or **congenitally missing teeth**. Parents often ask if these missing lateral incisors will ultimately need to be replaced with a bridge or implant, and the answer is Yes, because we need to develop the palate and dental arch for a balanced face and to create sufficient room for the tongue and to optimize structural space for optimal breathing.

These goals will create the space meant for the lateral incisors so that the missing teeth can be reinstated with artificial tooth replacements. Fortunately, with modern restorative technology, a beautiful, natural looking incisor can be constructed, and a good outcome can be assured; usually, the restorative phase is done in adulthood when growth is completed.

The permanent second bicuspids are also commonly congenitally missing. This is one good reason to have a PAN radiograph taken for a complete scan of the child's developing teeth. When detected early, it can inform the special need to preserve the deciduous tooth that is not going to be replaced.

Despite that a child may appear to have well aligned teeth, parents still need to keep a look out for other clues to growth deficiency. When growth of the midface and the upper jaw is hindered, the child may present with a **flat** or **concave facial profile**.

Classifications

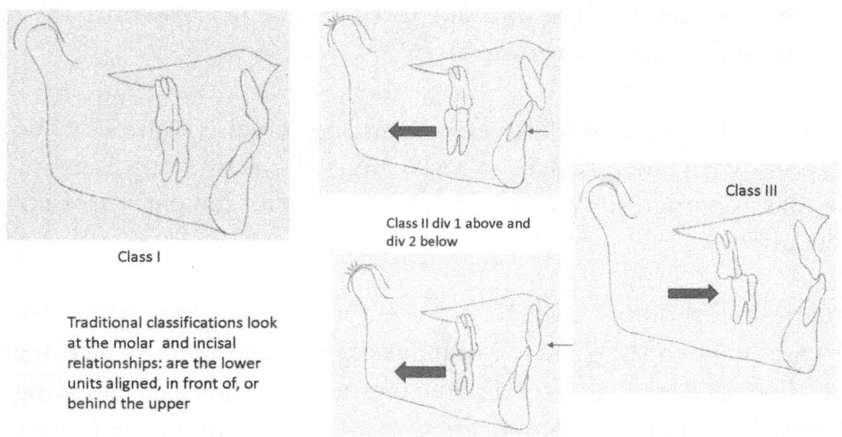
Class I
Class II div 1 above and div 2 below
Class III
Traditional classifications look at the molar and incisal relationships: are the lower units aligned, in front of, or behind the upper

Figure 28: Classification of occlusion.

Dentists generally refer to the following classification of occlusion.

- Class I: the upper jaw/teeth line up with the lower ones with optimal overbite and overjet of the front teeth. Facial profile is balanced. Note that Class I is not common in our modern world.
- Class II: the lower jaw/teeth are set back relative to the upper. This is further classified into divisions.

- » Class II Division 1: the permanent upper incisors are normally proclined. This is commonly a result of some myofunctional issue such as a tongue thrust or thumb-sucking habit that pushes the mandible back.
- » Class II Division 2: the permanent upper incisors are not proclined but lean back (retroclined) forming a smaller or flattened dental arch. The mandible is at risk of being pushed back. Class II division 2 occlusion often is associated with TMD and chronic headaches. The teeth will need active therapy to correct the incisor inclination.

- Class III: stronger mandible growth relative to the upper, with the lower jaw/teeth positioned forward to the upper ones. The maxilla may be undersized and set back relative to the cranium. The anterior teeth may be in cross-bite, or have little or no overjet.

Class II Division 2 and Class III are strong genetic traits. A child of parents with these classes of occlusion who shows any hints of these class characteristics should be investigated for early growth intervention.

Mothers tend to know best. If you are a mum and you suspect that your child may not be growing quite as expected in the jaw, face and teeth, then seek advice early. Early treatment is the easiest. Fixing problems later is more complicated, more expensive and may only give compromised results.

7

Max the Maxilla

Having read through all the chapters up to here, you will by now understand how important it is to ensure that your child's jaws develop correctly. Generally, jaw growth deficiency lies in the upper jaw.

Good Reasons for Maximising the Maxilla

1. To provide plenty of room for future permanent teeth to align and to lessen the need for any tooth extractions.

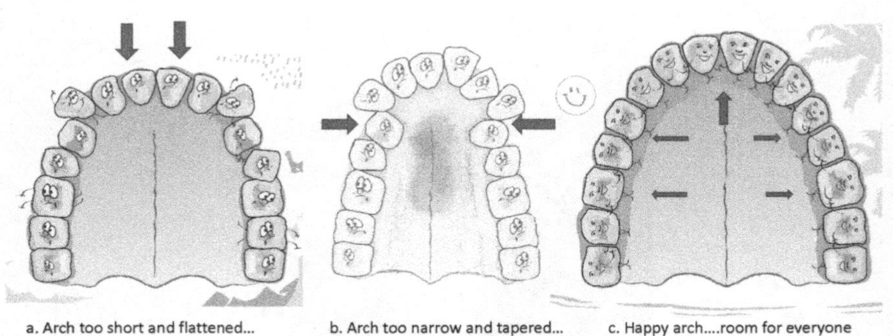

a. Arch too short and flattened...
b. Arch too narrow and tapered...
c. Happy arch....room for everyone

Figure 29: Undersized arch causes crowding.

2. To have a beautiful and broad smile. When teeth are removed and/ or dental arches are small, the results are often dark buccal corridors that detract from a smile. Wide dental arches will fill the smile with teeth displayed from one corner of the mouth to the other.

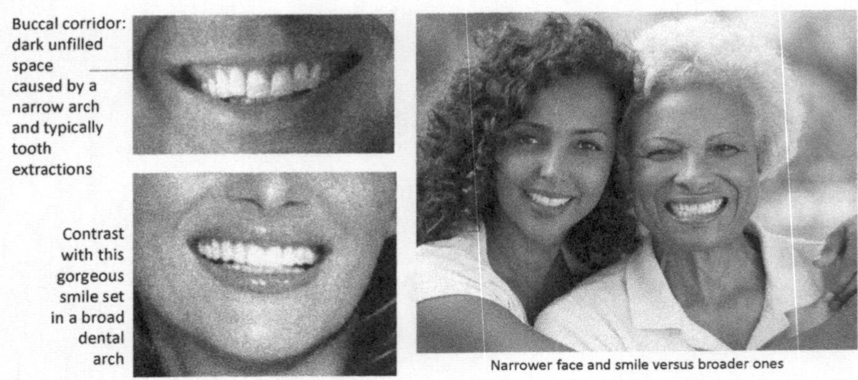

Buccal corridor: dark unfilled space caused by a narrow arch and typically tooth extractions
Contrast with this gorgeous smile set in a broad dental arch
Narrower face and smile versus broader ones

Figure 30: Broad and narrow smiles.

3. To accommodate the tongue. Often the tongue is too big for the mouth. You cannot shrink the tongue but you can develop the maxilla to accommodate it.

4. To not constrain but allow the mandible to develop forward during growth. Compression in the TMJs must be avoided to reduce the risk of TMD.

Do not constrain!!

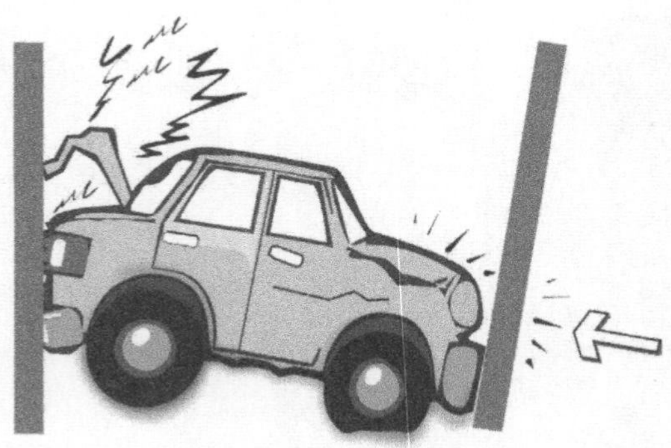

Figure 31

5. To support a wide nasal cavity which facilitates airflow and nasal breathing.

6. To develop a balanced and attractive facial profile by allowing nature to put the lower jaw where it needs to go as the head and midface grow forward.

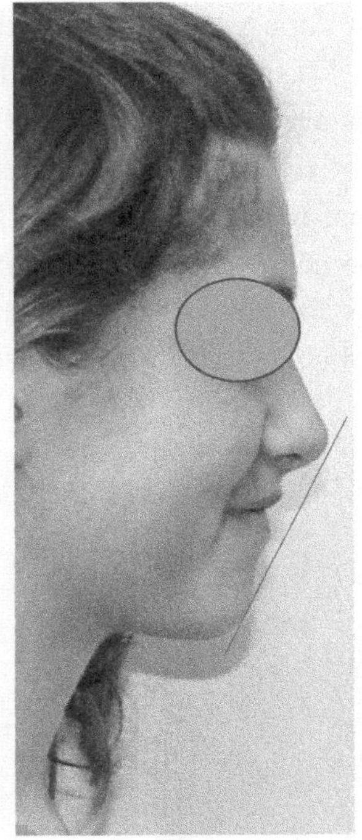

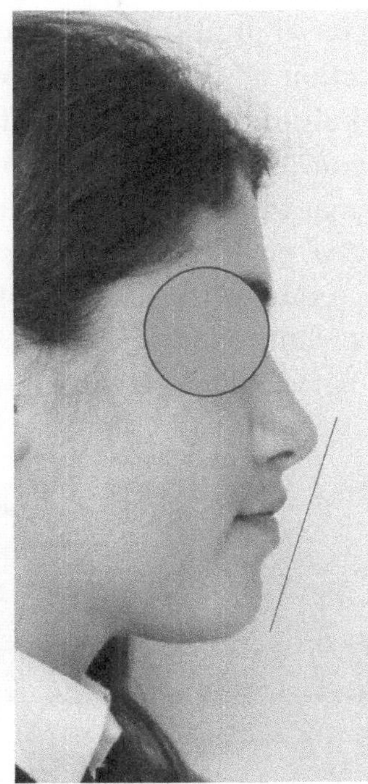

Figure 32: Facial profile improved after maxilla expansion.

Head X-rays: Why and When We Need Them

By the age of 7 years or even earlier as necessary, the child can have x-rays of the head and jaw taken. Dentists use these to analyse the direction that the jaws, face and teeth are growing.

The two useful ones are the orthopantomogram (OPG), also known as panoramic x-rays of the head, and the lateral cephalogram (or 'lat ceph') which are both 2D imaging.

The OPG will show if any teeth may be congenitally missing or if there may be supernumerary teeth present. These are extra teeth above the number that we normally have. It also helps detect any upper canines that may be at risk of being impacted (stuck) due to an undersized maxilla and shortage of space.

The lateral cephalogram which captures the side view of the head and facial profile can be traced, measured and analysed to assess the direction of the child's growth in this area. This analysis is called a **cephalometric analysis**. The measurements are made in relation to a frame of references and compared to a set of average values. There are many analyses taught and used. The ideal methods measure the relative position of the jaws against the base of the cranium to give us a guide to the position of the maxilla. As we have discussed it is important to know if the maxilla may be set back too far and growth guidance may need to be initiated.

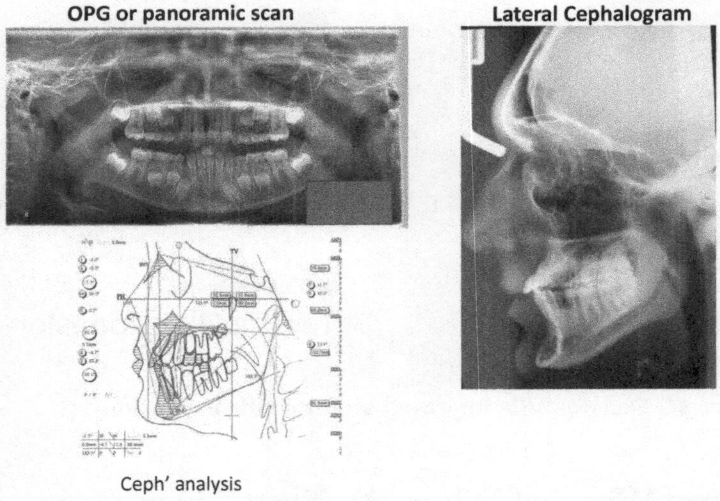

Figure 33: OPG and lateral ceph x-rays.

There is a new digital 3D imaging known as cone-beam volumetric tomographs (CBVT) which can provide 3D views of the cranium, jaw and teeth. As more of this type of x-ray equipment is developed and released on the market, they are able to provide better quality images with lower exposure to x-rays as well as at a lower cost for the patients. CBVT, due to their 3D imaging capability, are particularly helpful for studying the jaw joints, the nasal cavities, sinuses and the airway at the back of the throat.

There are many methods used by dentists to help develop the maxilla, but below are some common ones.

'Expanding' Appliances

If the maxilla needs to be expanded, or I prefer the term 'developed', then the dentist will prescribe dental or oral appliances (also referred to as 'plates') which are customised to fit the child's mouth.

The appliance is made to fit inside the palate of the child and this is to be worn for several months. These plates usually will have some screws or springs as components that need to be turned or 'activated' every few days. This activation expands the plate, which in turn will press and stimulate the maxilla to develop in the direction that we wish to gain extra growth in. For this reason, they are often known as orthopaedic appliances because they remodel or expand the bony structures to reshape the palate, and prepare and create space for the adult teeth to grow into.

There are myriads of expansion appliances designed by dentists over the years and used to achieve the orthopedic changes required.

Broadly speaking, the appliance needs to be worn full-time (24/7) for the activation to work satisfactorily and efficiently without relapses.

Removable Appliances have the advantage of being able to be removed for hygiene. However, their correct use will require good compliance by the child and good support and supervision by the parents.

They are removed from the mouth only for cleaning purposes and for activation. As the plate is widened, so will the maxilla as it is gently nudged along. In my experience, the younger patients are usually the most cooperative or adaptive to wearing these appliances. I have made appliances for patients as young as 4 years old with great results.

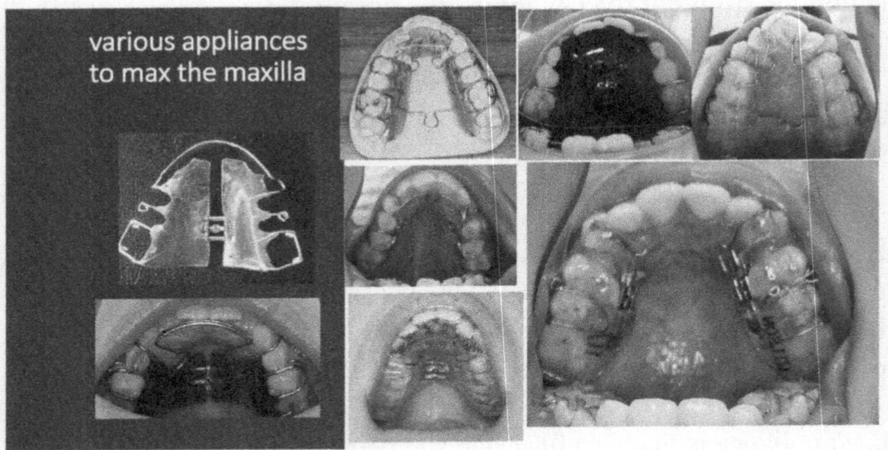

Figure 34: Appliances.

Fixed Appliances are bonded to selected teeth and cannot be removed during the whole duration of treatment. They have the advantage of staying inside the mouth full-time for improved and controlled activation. However, mouth and teeth hygiene during the use of these appliances can be a challenge as they cannot be taken out for cleaning. Fortunately, these days new dental hygiene tools such as air or water jet spray cleaners are available and help make the task easier.

Forward-pull Face Mask

The forward-pull face mask, also referred to as a 'reversed' head gear, is a frame that fits around the child's face and provides the attachments for elastic bands to **protract the maxilla forward**. It is used in conjunction with a palate expansion appliance and is worn mostly during the evening and night. Please be aware that this is not the usual headgear that we commonly see teenagers wear to *retract* their upper teeth backwards, against growth.

Forward-pull face mask are used in the very young for maximum effectiveness. Ideally, they are prescribed for those between 4–6 years old because that is when bones are very adaptable, and again to nip growth issues at the bud. Despite its appearance, I find that young kids are cooperative with wearing a forward-pull mask, especially when the parents are helpful in supervising its proper use.

Two types of forward pull face mask, or reversed headgear

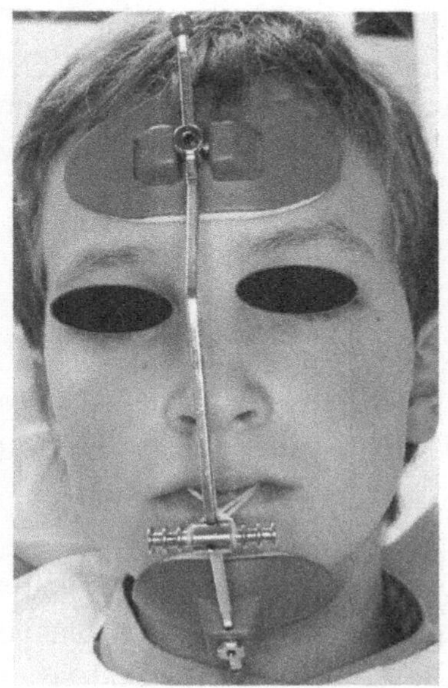

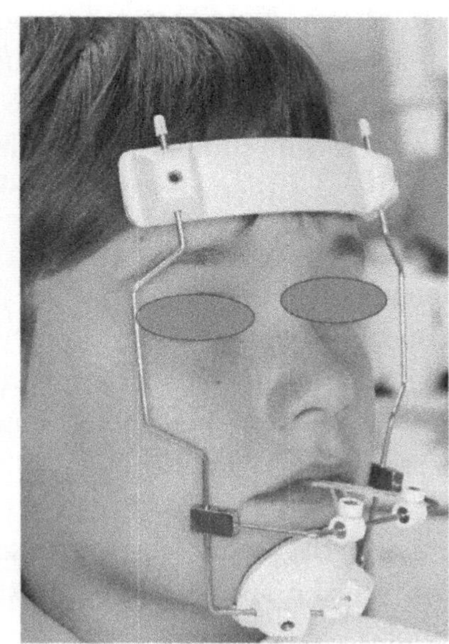

Figure 35: Face mask.

Orthognathic Surgery

These are surgical techniques to treat a young adult when growth is finished (typically in the late teens), or later. Parts of the upper or lower jaw or both may be sectioned and moved to correct shape, dimension and alignment.

Again, there are pros and cons which, like all surgical treatment, need to be fully understood and taken into consideration by the patient and parents. This procedure may be avoided if growth problems are picked up and intercepted early.

Functional Issues

We refer to the group of related issues such as mouth breathing, poor muscle posture or aberrant tongue habits that contribute to the structural deficiency as **functional issues** and these obviously cannot be ignored. For the best outcomes, treatment maximising the maxilla structure will need to be accompanied by various functional therapy either before, during or after the maxilla development.

There can be some confusion with the term 'functional' in this area of dentistry. Note that a 'functional appliance' can also refer to an oral appliance that is prescribed for a child with a retruded mandible that needs to be developed more forward once the maxilla has been expanded. The common removable functional appliances include the Twin Blocks, Bionator and the Biobloc III.

Orofacial Myology

Orofacial Myology (OFM) or Oral Myofunctional Therapy (OMT) are health disciplines that are involved with training the muscles of the jaws and mouth for improved functioning and correcting aberrant tongue habits.

Just as orthopaedic surgery treating other parts of the body calls upon physiotherapy and exercises to promote healing, dentofacial orthopaedic changes such as maxilla development or orthodontics will be more effective when the associated muscles are retrained to function optimally as well.

OFM is a natural and essential process of guiding a child's growth for a beautiful and healthy set of teeth, jaws, head, face and airway.

I first heard of OFM in the late 1980s when Dr John Mew, a British orthodontist (specialist) and founder of the **orthotropic premise**, came out from the UK to teach his techniques to a handful of general dentists here in Melbourne. He stressed that for an effective treatment outcome, there is a need for the patient to learn to keep their mouth closed and tongue properly postured.

Mew wrote an amazing book titled *Biobloc Therapy* about his treatment philosophy and maxilla expansion technique – 'the thoughts that initiated it, the research that founded it and the clinical work that developed it …' – and each time I pick up the book to read, I feel enormous admiration for and inspiration from his wisdom and passion on the subject.

OFM was such an unknown subject back then and, for many years to follow, few dentists understood why or how to apply any of these exercises for the benefit of their patients.

Fortunately, this important subject has now gained wider recognition, and education in this area is gaining momentum and included in many worthwhile dental health symposium programs around the world. There are, however, too few dedicated OFM therapists in Australia currently.[24]

Typically, an oral myofunctional therapist (OMT) may be a speech pathologist, a dental therapist or hygienist who has undergone further training in the subject. Dentists and osteo- or chiro-practitioners also take these courses to learn how to detect unhelpful muscle patterns and habits that may interfere with treatment, and how appropriate exercises can be included as part of the therapy for their patients.

A course of dedicated OM Therapy may run for a few weeks. Ideally, they should be introduced to complement a course of dentofacial growth guidance and breathing retraining. These exercises aim to achieve the Big 3 as discussed earlier.

I have noticed that some proactive ENT surgeons are also including OMT as part of their patient care. We should not be surprised because in order to improve breathing and airway issues, patients must use the muscles of the face and mouth correctly.

---

24. For more information, visit: Academy of Orofacial Myofunctional Therapy (AOMT) at https://aomtinfo.org/ and The Australian Association of Orofacial Myology (AOMT) at http://australianassociationoforofacialmyology.org.au/

Role of Genetics

Are small maxilla and/or retruded mandible inherited? Parents often comment that the poor child takes after one of the parents and erroneously believe that nothing can be done to correct the situation.

Although genetic influence does play a role (especially in the Class III strong mandible pattern and the Class II Division 2 short maxilla pattern), we can see that there are many 'environmental' influences that are within the control of the parents to mitigate, in order to redirect growth in the right direction

So, one may ask what is causing this avalanche of relative underdevelopment of the upper jaw in our modern world? There are several theories offered by dentists, anthropologists, biologists and their published books are certainly well worth reading.[25,26,27,28] The consensus points to mouth breathing, poor airway and sleep, poor use of orofacial muscles and making the wrong food choice. We are selecting to eat more processed foods, and this includes baby formula for infants. These types of food are often made to be eaten fast and easily without involving much chewing effort, and often with no consideration for the nutritious content.

An analogy is a child who never had to walk or to exercise the legs but was carried everywhere. The child's leg muscles would atrophy. As we no longer eat harder and tougher foods, our orofacial muscles are not properly used and the skeletal structures they connect to do not develop as they should.

Orthodontic Teeth Alignment

Once optimal dentofacial growth has been achieved and functional issues controlled, then usually the permanent teeth will come out perfectly with no need for further treatment as nature intended.

---

25. WA Price, *Nutrition and Physical Degeneration*, Price-Pottinger, 1939
26. R Corruccni, *How Anthropology Informs the Orthodontic Diagnosis of Malocclusion's Causes*, Edwin Mellen Press, 1999
27. A Fonder, *The Dental Physician* (2nd Ed.), Medical-Dental Arts, 1985
28. DE Lieberman, *The Story of the Human Body*, Vintage Books, 2013

However, sometimes it may be desirable at this stage for the young adult to have the teeth alignment idealised and this is where braces or newer techniques such as clear aligners can be used. These are treatment techniques that can fine-tune the alignment, the inclination, and/or rotation of the individual tooth. Orthodontists are especially skilled in this phase of therapy.

Adjunct Complementary Therapy

I have also found that treatment provided to my patient by osteopaths and/or chiro-practitioners who specialise in the fields of the cranium and jaw can enhance my treatment outcome for the child. These practitioners take care of the neural system to ensure good connectivity between the various parts of the body that impact on the growing dentofacial structures.

The conclusion is that your dentist and practitioners from various health disciplines must collaborate to treat the child as a whole patient, and not just the teeth, for a successful outcome

Burnout?

Parents often ask me, 'Is my child too young for treatment, or will my child get burnt out if we start at such a young age?' This thought is often also used as a criticism from opponents to the philosophy of treating early.

My opinion based on observation of my patients is that treating the young is a lot easier, because the problem is not so ingrained. The child is still growing and the skeletal structure is adaptable. As we all appreciate, bad habits that are well set is much harder to undo. We certainly cannot sit and watch the child suffer from poor airway, sleep and growth.

As mentioned before, scientific studies are increasingly finding that maximising the growth of the maxilla can help treat other significant medical conditions in children such as SDB, OSA, ear infections and nocturnal bedwetting.

Indirectly, it has also been found now to be linked to childhood obesity, childhood behavioural and social issues, and learning issues paralleling those observed in ADHD.

However, I stress that for a successful outcome, parents must be enrolled and dedicated to helping the child grow the maxilla to the max and supervise the breathing and orofacial muscle retraining (daily exercises). This is an area I often find that parents, in our modern and busy world, let us down.

What Happens When the Dental Arches Shrink?

Here I want to share with the reader the case of a young oriental adult who I was sitting next to for several days at a publishing workshop.

When he heard that I was a dentist, he commented that he had just been paying big sums of money for his dental treatment. He was also suffering from TMD with clicking and painful TMJs during that conference.

I noted he had a flattened midface and a long face shape, and I said to him that perhaps his mandible and tongue are constrained by an undersized and set-back maxilla. His response was interesting.

He said, 'Ah ha, that makes so much sense because ever since I had eight teeth removed with my orthodontic treatment, to have my remaining teeth straightened, my tongue has felt cramped and uncomfortable. I hate how my tongue sits nowadays. It's like it doesn't know where it belongs.'

Beware of the collateral unwanted outcome of losing tongue space and airway when aiming for straight teeth at all cost.

This young man is not alone, and his experience is in fact sadly common based on what I find in my patients who attend my practice for TMD pain treatment and occlusion rehabilitation.

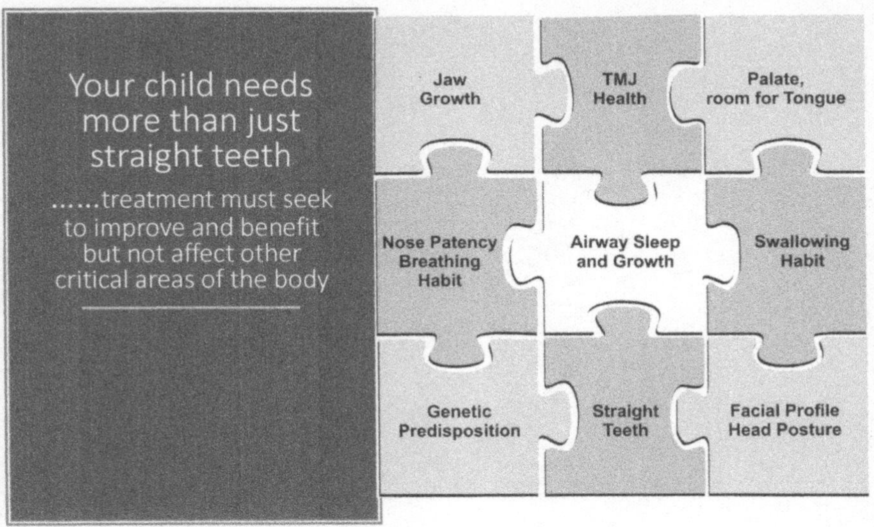

Figure 36: Jig-saw of the bigger picture.

8

A Pain-free Life

In this chapter, I want to show the reader some typical adult patient cases that I have treated for jaw and tooth problems and pain who also have small maxilla, poor jaw alignment and a compromised pharyngeal airway. Name initials are used here to protect the identity of the persons.

FO's Narrow Maxilla and TMD Pain

FO is a 30-year-old female with chronic and debilitating jaw and facial pain and limitation of jaw opening/closing. She had done a circuit of seeing medical doctors and had taken pain medications. She had been treated by several physical therapists for a period of 8 months but the symptoms continued to affect her daily life and work as a social worker.

A comprehensive study of her teeth, jaw, head and facial muscles which included CBVT imaging of her jaw joints and a sleep test found that she had set back maxilla and mandible, compressed TMJs and oxygen desaturation during sleep with a sleep disturbance index higher than is considered acceptable. She was observed to have a mouth-breathing habit and she was not aware of the importance of breathing through her nose.

FO in fact had orthodontic treatment in her teens whereby eight permanent teeth had been removed, leaving her with a small maxilla and a lower jaw that was held back.

After her jaw pain symptoms were treated with dental splints, she had chosen to have a second course of orthodontic treatment but this time with the goal of widening her maxilla and bringing her jaws more forward to correct the problems and to provide a longer-term resolution.

Some of the teeth that were extracted in her teens have now been replaced with artificial teeth (and implants) that can fit in the treated and wider dental arch.

She has learned the importance of the Big 3 and she now breathes and sleeps better. The whole series of treatment took several years to complete and presented a significant financial challenge for FO. It was also difficult to take time off work for the treatment.

MK's Narrow Maxilla and TMD Pain

MK is a 56-year-old female with jaw and facial pain, tooth sensitivity, sleeping problems and depression. She had been seeing medical doctors and specialists, counsellors, physical therapists and taken significant amounts of different medication to control the above symptoms.

MK had orthodontic treatment during her teenage years when four premolar teeth were removed, and the remaining teeth aligned. A few years later, her wisdom teeth were removed as well. Having lost eight of her adult teeth meant that the remaining 24 now appeared well lined up, albeit in smaller dental arches. Though her teeth were reasonably straight, the upper and lower jaws were not relating well and her TMJs were compressed.

A comprehensive study and analysis of her teeth, occlusion, TMJs, facial profile, breathing habits and sleep concluded that MK still has narrow dental arches, inadequate tongue space, set back jaws, compressed TMJs and nightly sleep disturbance that may be attributed to choking. MK was habitually breathing through her mouth and had incorrect tongue posture away from her palate.

Initial treatment with dental splints were successful in improving most of her pain symptoms. She is now considering yet another course of orthodontic treatment, possibly in conjunction with surgery, to maximise her maxilla and to allow the mandible to track more forward and enable her tongue to posture correctly. The aim is to improve her airway so that she can breathe and sleep better.

The splint therapy and a planned second round of orthodontic treatment to attempt to max her maxilla will be setting her back several tens of thousands of dollars. She will also have to have the extracted teeth replaced in the finally treated dental arches. Without this course of treatment to provide more oral space she is likely to continue with TMJ pain, sleep deprivation and debilitation for the rest of her life.

CW's TMD Pain and Headaches, Class III with Short Maxilla

CW is a 35-year-old male floor manager for a busy industrial firm and was referred to me by his physical therapist who had been treating him for chronic and debilitating jaw and facial pain. He reported that he had been suffering with pain in the jaw area for over 10 years. Physical therapy and medication had provided only temporary relief.

CW's teeth were sound with no cavity. His dental history included four years of orthodontic treatment in his late teens to correct a prominent and crooked appearance of his upper incisors. He recalled having to use some head-gear with elastic force to pull the upper-front teeth back. At the end of the orthodontic therapy, he had four wisdom teeth removed under general anesthesia due to lack of space in his dental arches

A comprehensive study and analysis of CW's teeth and jaw showed that he has small dental arches that can accommodate only 28 out of the full complement of 32 teeth. Although his teeth were reasonably straight, the maxilla was short lengthwise and the mandible was trapped. His left-side TMJ was compressed. He also snored, and clenched and grinded his teeth in his sleep. A sleep study conducted showed reduced oxygen saturation and a high index of sleep disturbance. CW habitually breathed through his mouth.

Splint therapy that repositioned his mandible has been able to provide significant symptom relief for CW but is a great inconvenience for him due to the interference with his speech that is important in his work. For a longer-term resolution, he is considering treatment to max his maxilla to free the mandible and TMJs, and to provide more oral space for his tongue and to improve pharyngeal airway.

This planned course of treatment will present a financial and time challenge for CW at this stage of his life as he must take into consideration his situation at work and his young family.

OT's Class III, Chronic TMD, Back Pain, Bruxing and Broken Teeth

OT is a 57-year-old male. This patient has 12 missing teeth from his mouth. He has lost these teeth one by one over the years due to the stress and breakage from perpetual and severe clenching and grinding. Whilst there is insignificant crowding of his remaining 24 teeth, his upper dental arch is small and his upper and lower jaws are mismatched. He is a chronic mouth breather.

OT has a Class III occlusion with the lower arch constrained by a smaller upper dental arch. Though this discrepancy is not obvious, it is enough to have put pressure on the condyles, and insufficient space for his tongue. He reported symptoms of chronic jaw pain, headaches, neck and back pain, and poor-quality sleep all his adult life. He routinely sees physical therapists for pain relief.

Although his teeth can be repaired, he would ideally need to have upper dental arch made wider and brought more forward, his occlusion repositioned to provide improved support for his TMJs and increased oral space for his tongue so that his airway during sleep is optimal which will give him sound quality sleep.

However, he is now at a stage in his life that to consider the comprehensive but optimal treatment plan to rid his jaw pains is out of reach. Therefore, it is expected that as time goes by he will continue to suffer gradual breakdown and loss of the remaining teeth, one by one, despite the best restorative repair he can afford. It is also likely that he will continue to suffer the various chronic pains.

NI's Deep Overbite, Retruded jaw and OSA

NI is an 80-year-old female who has lost half her teeth. Her remaining teeth are slightly crooked but presented as a deep overbite, collapsed support for her TMJs, a constrained tongue and she uses a Continuous Positive Air Pressure (CPAP) every night to treat OSA.

I still offered her a comprehensive and doable treatment plan because I wanted to help her rehabilitate her teeth and mouth so that she can eat and enjoy her food, to obtain the necessary nutrients right up to her last meal. Apart from restoring her dentition, I also initiated a conversation about correct orofacial muscle patterns and the all-essential function of nasal breathing during waking hours and sleep.

I knew that once she can eat well, breathe well and sleep better, she would be in a much better position to tackle other degenerative conditions that she has. Perhaps the extensive treatment plan that I had carried out for her might not have been necessary had she received good dental growth guidance from a young age.

In fact, the many thousands of dollars that she was spending on dental restorations and dentures at her age might have been put to more advantageous use much earlier, as an investment for a lifelong enjoyment of having a full complement of sound and healthy teeth, good occlusion, forward jaws, good airway and sleep. Perhaps the CPAP unit that she is using now might not be necessary, nor the medication for reflux that she has been taking for the last couple of years.

The above examples show how a majority of my adult patients with symptoms of tooth breakdown from bruxing share the common characteristics of an undersized maxilla, poor breathing habit, inadequate room for the tongue, sleep disordered breathing and poor sleep. About 60% even had a history of past orthodontic treatment that simply treated their crooked teeth by removing sound teeth but had not addressed these other related factors in a bigger, total-health paradigm.

It is challenging to help these patients as their symptoms are advanced.

The more effective approach would have been to begin from the beginning, to initiate proper jaw growth in the newborn and to pay attention to the child's breathing early. This approach will mitigate many chronic pains relating to the jaws throughout life. The bonus is that with a properly developed maxilla, and with correct habits such as the Big 3 in place, the teeth will naturally align well, giving the child a broad and beautiful smile for life.

Of course, there could be other causes of TMD such as trauma and injury from accidents and other chronic systemic illnesses such as arthritis which, of course, must be taken into consideration in treatment planning.

9

Key to Health

As I studied my notes collected from past seminars and courses over the years, and as I searched my ever-growing collection of books, I rediscovered an amazing book which I must share with the reader. This book called *The Breath of Life or Mal-respiration and its Effects Upon the Enjoyments and Life of Man* (also titled *Shut Your Mouth and Save Your Life*) was written in the mid-1800s by American author George Catlin (1796-1872).

Catlin was by profession a lawyer and a portrait painter. Later in life, he travelled in the western plains of North and South America to live with, paint and study the Native American Indian tribes in their natural communities and habitat. He apparently visited many tribes, a total of about two million natives. Thus, he had an opportunity to observe and compare the way of life, especially in the area of health and diseases, of the Native Americans with that of his own background.

At that time, he was aware that the average life span in the so-called 'civilised' communities he came from was less than one-fifth of the expected life of 70 years (3 scores plus 10), and the prevalence of infant mortality was high.

He was astonished to learn that by contrast the various tribal natives covering a large span of the America continent were altogether a much healthier people despite their more basic living conditions.

There was no parallel to the rate of child mortality that was seen in the civilised world.

There were less premature deaths, and significantly less incidences of mental and physical 'deformities' as they were known then.

He became curious as to why the difference existed, and what was causing the breakdown of health and the magnitude of diseases in the 'civilised' world but not in the other. He searched for answers by observation and talking with the natives.

First, he observed that the native's diet consisted mainly of locally wild-caught fish, buffalo meat, venison, maize and vegetables.

After years of observation, he concluded that the cause of ill health amongst his own civilised people was quite simply a neglect to secure a good night's sleep, supported by proper breathing through the nose. He wrote that quiet and natural sleep is the physician and the restorer of mankind and animals.[29]

He noted how a native mother at the end of a breastfeed would lower the infant to sleep and be sure to press its lips together to keep the mouth closed.

By contrast, he observed that most children in more civilised communities inside their sanitised homes comforted by heating and cooling, in fact slept with their mouth open.

Catlin, in the mid-1800s, had said that nature has given us such a sophisticated organ as the nose to ensure that air is well purified before it reaches our lung, yet man is so unwise to not use the nose but instead the mouth, to breathe. According to George Catlin keeping the mouth closed when breathing is the key to health.

29. G Catlin, *The Breath of Life*, USA, John Wiley & Son, 1872, p.15.

I highly recommend this short book which contains interesting illustrations drawn by the author himself.

Drawing by George Catlin about 1860, comparing a group of children who mouth-breathed with another who kept their mouth closed……

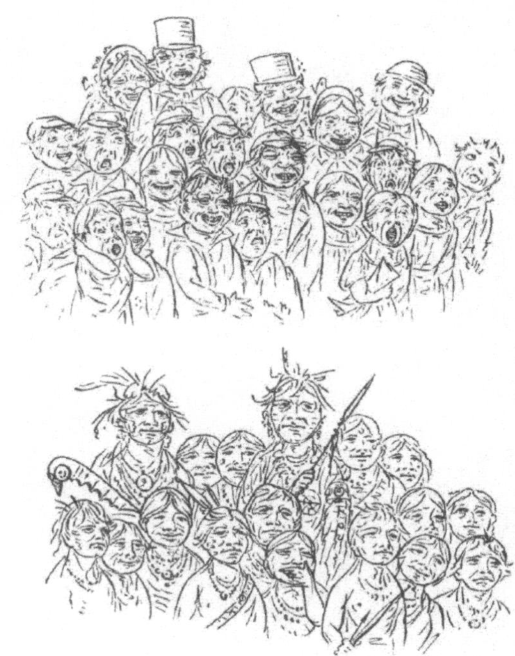

Figure 37: *The Breath of Life* **by George Catlin.**

10

Fast Forward

I believe that we can realistically look forward to a future where everyone has amazing teeth, gorgeously bright smiles with great looking faces, balanced occlusion that keeps the TMJs healthy, and broad jaws that do not constrain the tongue – a future where everyone breathes well, sleeps well, and lives a life free of chronic pain.

People will be happier as there will be less suffering from dental and other related chronic health issues. Paying the dentist's bill will take on a different meaning and may not be such dirty words. It would be a future with a much shorter queue for medical and hospital care, and the budget for dental and medical health can be greatly reduced.

I hope that the reader can see the big picture that I do and that it begins with paying early attention to guiding your child's dentofacial growth in the right direction.

I think we may also need a paradigm shift at our teaching institutions. We need our university and dental schools to educate dental undergraduates on the wider paradigm of dental health care and its broader links to other professional health areas.

Education is the key, not just for the health professionals but also for the community at large at all levels. Parents, grandparents, carers and extended family attending to a child need to work together in an integrative manner, and consider the paradigm discussed in this book.

The body is not compartmentalised into isolated parts. Quite the contrary, nature is awesome at creating this amazing body of ours that consists of many physiology systems which all connect and work together perfectly. We need to understand how the function or dysfunction of one system can affect the others and attempt to address the root cause of a dysfunction for a positive outcome for the whole body rather than just treating the isolated symptoms.

All health professionals from various disciplines need to embrace the paradigm shift and work together more closely for the benefit of the patient's wellbeing.

We also need the health funds to take part in this paradigm shift. Restorative treatments are still preferential for claiming benefits. Health benefit payouts for preventative therapy including health education has always been appalling or non-existent. This must change. They must be prepared to support the professionals and their clients, the fund members, and pay benefits for fees charged for time well spent by professionals in educating patients.

Epilogue

The longer I have been in practice, the stronger my conclusion that a typical dentist's routine of helping to repair broken down teeth or restore hopeless occlusion is too much hard work. It is very challenging for the dentist, very costly for the patient and often yields only a compromised result. It is not the optimal way of going about improving dental health. There has to be a better way, and there is a better way. Therefore, I decided it was time I shared my thoughts.

As I began to write this book, I came to realise, and panicked somewhat, that I cannot condense every bit of what I have learned over the decades of clinical practice and continuing education into a book of this size. It has been a challenge to decide which bit of knowledge would be the most essential and useful in relation to growing beautiful teeth. I hope that I managed to explain with just the right amount of detail to make the points clear enough so as not to confuse.

This book can serve as a beginner's guide to growing beautiful teeth for one's child. Much more is now available out there on the internet. I am hoping that once parents understand the simple but essential basics as discussed in this book, they can research further to expand their knowledge on this interesting subject of dentofacial growth.

The steps to take are simple but it takes dedication and courage to do it differently. Do not wait to see how far a problem will pan out and hope that someone can fix it later. The change from a fix-it-later attitude to nipping it at the buds, to nurture growth and mitigate the problem is the paradigm shift that both the parents and the professionals need to strive for.

Unless we make the change, nothing will change.

Acknowledgements

Deep gratitude and thanks are due to my husband Bo Norlin for his encouragement and support with this project and for supplying humour when needed;

to all my patients past and present for their trust and confidence in my care; to the models in Figure 10: newborns Alicia, Ayla, Anya, Hannah, Harrison, Mia, and Oscar, and their mums for permission to use their photos; to Natasa Denman for planting the seed that led to the outcome of this book, and BusyBird Publishing for their help in book production; to Vivien Fowler my practice assistant for her help in every way that she could possibly give; to Irene Sajn of iDraw4U for her help with some of the illustrations; to all my friends far and near for their patience and support whilst I kept away to write.

Thanks to all the exceptional Gurus I have the good fortune of learning from (listed on my practice website www.princessdental.com.au); and to my colleagues, "the usual suspects", whom I meet at endless professional courses and meetings, for their friendship and support in our educational journey together.

About the author ...

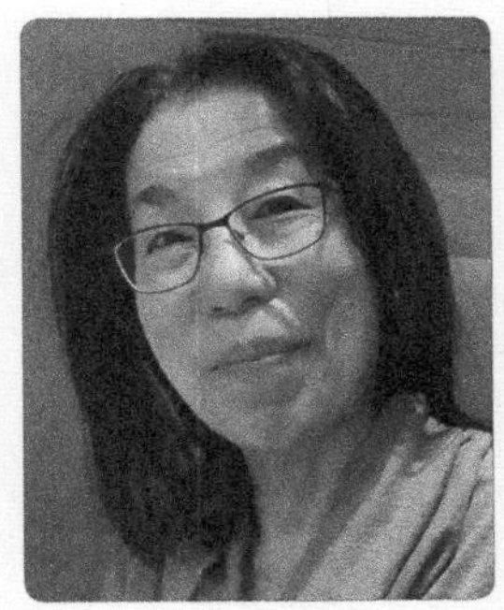

Born in SE Asia, Estie Bav migrated to Australia when she was 16. She finished high school in Geraldton and Perth, then graduated with a Bachelor of Dental Science from the University of Western Australia. Earlier in her career she served in the Royal Australian Air Force as a Squadron Leader senior dental officer.

In 1991 Estie co-established Princess Street Dental Group in Kew, City of Melbourne, where she has continued practising as a general dentist (www.princessdental.com.au).

She is a member of the Australian Dental Association, the American Academy of Craniofacial Pain, American Academy of Physiological Medicine and Dentistry, the Australian Medical Laser Association, and a member and certified senior instructor of the International Association for Orthodontics.

She can be reached at **estie@drestiebav.com**

Glossary

ADHD
Attention Deficit Hyperactive Disorder.

adult teeth
Permanent teeth or second set of teeth (which comes out after the primary teeth, also referred to as deciduous teeth, milk teeth or baby teeth).

anterior
Of or near the front (e.g. anterior teeth), opposite to posterior.

baby teeth
Deciduous teeth or first set of teeth, also referred to as milk teeth or primary teeth.

bicuspid
Another term for premolar, the smaller back tooth between the canine (or cuspid) and the molar.

bite
How the bottom teeth close up against the top teeth. The dental term is occlusion.

bruxing
Clenching and grinding of teeth, usually involuntarily and during sleep, which can lead to severe wear or breakage of teeth.

buccal
Of the cheek, facing the cheek, or referring to a position on the cheek side e.g. buccal surface of a tooth.

buccal corridor
The dark space seen at the sides of the mouth when one smiles, caused by a narrow dental arch that inadequately fills in the space inside the cheeks.

CBVT
Cone Beam Volumetric Tomograph: 3D digital imaging of the head and jaw area using x-rays.

ceph analysis
Tracing of the head, face and jaw structures of a side-view head x-ray. These are measured in linear and angle measurements from a frame of reference and then checked against a set of known data to assess the relative position of the jaws.

condyle
Anatomical structure: the two knobbly ends of the lower jaw bone. The condyles connect the lower jaw to the base of the skull.

CPAP
Continuous Positive Air Pressure: a small compressor to pump air and facilitate breathing via a hose and a nose-piece. It is used to treat OSA.

craniofacial
Of the skull and face structure.

cranium
The skull structure that holds the brain.

crossbite
Malocclusion where the upper teeth bite inside to the lower teeth. Crossbites may be at the front of the dental arch (anterior crossbite) or at the back (posterior crossbite).

cuspid
Another name for the canine or tooth number three in each quadrant. (See quadrant.)

deciduous teeth
Primary teeth or first set of teeth, also referred to as milk teeth or baby teeth.

dental arch
The arch formed by the lined-up teeth in the upper or the lower jaw.

dentofacial
Of the teeth and face, this is commonly used in the treatment paradigm referred to in this book.

distal
The side furthest away from the midline of the jaw. Usually referring to the 'back' of the mouth. (Opposite to mesial).

ENT surgeon
Ear, Nose and Throat surgeon.

enuresis (nocturnal enuresis)
involuntary urination (during the night).

erupt
Referring to new teeth when coming out through the gums.

facial profile
Outline of the face as seen from the side.

frenulectomy
Minor surgical procedure to release a tied tongue.

frenulum or frenum, lingual
Oral tissues that tether the underside of the tongue to the floor of the mouth, also called tethered oral tissues or TOT.

frenulum or frenum, labial
Thickened rope of oral tissues that tether the inside of the lip to the alveolar bone near the front teeth.

impacted teeth
The (adult) teeth that are not erupted but remain in the jaw bone, usually due to crowding and lack of space.

labial
Of or relating to the lip; the side facing the lip.

lateral incisors
Front teeth that are to the side of the central teeth. The second tooth counting from the midline.

lingual
Of or relating to the tongue; the side facing the tongue.

lower jaw
Mandible.

malocclusion
Bad occlusion or dysfunctional bite.

mandibular
Of the mandible; that is, related to the lower jaw.

maxilla
Upper jaw, also referred to as the palate.

maxillary
Of the maxilla; that is, related to the upper jaw.

mesial
The side towards the midline of the jaw or the forward side of the jaw. (Opposite to distal).

mixed dentition
The stage when both primary and secondary dentition are present, during the transition as adult teeth are gradually replacing the milk teeth (approximately between 6 and 12 years of age).

occlusion
The way the lower teeth close up against the upper teeth.

occlusal reconstruction
An overhaul of one's teeth to optimise matching together of bottom teeth to top teeth, usually with crowns, bridges or dentures if significant numbers of teeth are missing.

occlusal rehabilitation
Another term for occlusal reconstruction.

OFM
Orofacial Myology, a health discipline involved with training the muscles of the jaws and mouth especially the tongue for improved function and habits.

OFMT
Orofacial Myotherapy. See OFM.

OPG
Orthopantomography, a panoramic x-ray scan of the jaws and teeth.

orthodontics / orthopedics
Dental treatment that aims at moving teeth to improve alignment using a system of wire and brackets attached to teeth (commonly known as braces). Orthopedics in this context refers to developing the bony jaw structure, guiding growth, creating space, in preparation for orthodontics.

orthognathic
Straightening of the jaw, used in reference to surgery that realigns a sectioned jaw.

OSA
Obstructive Sleep Apnea: a health condition whereby air intake is interrupted during sleep due to narrowing and obstruction in the upper airway.

PAN
Panaoramic x-ray scanning, also known as an OPG.

permanent teeth
Adult teeth or secondary teeth (which comes after the primary teeth, also referred to as deciduous teeth, milk teeth or baby teeth).

posterior
Of or near the back (e.g. back teeth), opposite of anterior.

premolar
The smaller of the back teeth that are positioned in front of the molar teeth, after the canines. Also known as a bicuspid.

primary teeth
Deciduous teeth or first set of teeth, also referred to as milk teeth or baby teeth.

profile (of the face)
The view of a face (especially the outline) from the side. See facial profile.

quadrant
A positional term describing where teeth are, i.e. upper right quadrant, upper left quadrant, lower left quadrant and lower right quadrant. Quadrants are also numbered 1st, 2nd, 3rd, 4th in the above order to make description simpler.

REM
Rapid Eye Movement, a later phase in the sleep cycle.

relapse
A return to the pre-treatment condition.

retruded

Referring to a position of the mandible that is further back relative to the maxilla or base of the cranium.

sagittal

Of the length from back to front, as opposed to the transverse width when referring to dental arch dimensions. Thus, sagittal development means developing forward.

SDB

Sleep Disordered Breathing.

secondary teeth

Adult teeth or permanent teeth (which comes out after the primary teeth, also referred to as deciduous teeth, milk teeth or baby teeth).

sleep physician

A doctor who specialises in sleep disorders.

T&A

Tonsillectomy and Adenoidectomy: surgical procedures to remove infected and/or enlarged tonsils and adenoids at the back of the throat.

TMD

Temporomandibular Dysfunction or Disorder – that is, problems in the jaw-joints.

TMJ

Temporomandibular Joint, or jaw joint, of which we each have two.

TOT

Tethered Oral Tissues, also known as a tongue-tie or ankyloglossia.

transverse

Referring to the width of the dental arch, and even the cranium.

unilateral

One side. Bilateral means both sides.

Additional Resources

P. McKeown, *Close Your Mouth*, ButeykoClinic.com, 2004

P. McKeown, *Buteyko Meets Dr. Mew*, ButeykoClinic.com, 2010

D.C. Page, *Your Jaws Your Life*, SmilePage Publishing, 2003

P. J. Ameisen, *Every Breath You Take*, New Holland Publishers, 1997

P. McKeown, *The Oxygen Advantage*, HarpersCollins, 2015

Notes

Notes

Notes